Alternative Approaches for Expanding the Air Force's Task Force True North Program

AGNES GEREBEN SCHAEFER, JOHN A. AUSINK, THOMAS GOUGHNOUR,
KRISTIE L. GORE, KIMBERLY JACKSON, PAUL EMSLIE

Prepared for the Department of the Air Force
Approved for public release; distribution unlimited

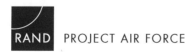

RAND PROJECT AIR FORCE

For more information on this publication, visit **www.rand.org/t/RRA269-1**.

About RAND

The RAND Corporation is a research organization that develops solutions to public policy challenges to help make communities throughout the world safer and more secure, healthier and more prosperous. RAND is nonprofit, nonpartisan, and committed to the public interest. To learn more about RAND, visit www.rand.org.

Research Integrity

Our mission to help improve policy and decisionmaking through research and analysis is enabled through our core values of quality and objectivity and our unwavering commitment to the highest level of integrity and ethical behavior. To help ensure our research and analysis are rigorous, objective, and nonpartisan, we subject our research publications to a robust and exacting quality-assurance process; avoid both the appearance and reality of financial and other conflicts of interest through staff training, project screening, and a policy of mandatory disclosure; and pursue transparency in our research engagements through our commitment to the open publication of our research findings and recommendations, disclosure of the source of funding of published research, and policies to ensure intellectual independence. For more information, visit www.rand.org/about/research-integrity.

RAND's publications do not necessarily reflect the opinions of its research clients and sponsors.

About This Report

The Vice Chief of Staff of the Air Force chartered the Task Force True North (TFTN) in December 2016. The objective of the task force is to "address seams/shortfalls with existing resources in order to more effectively enhance Airmen well-being and resilience and decrease negative outcomes such as interpersonal and self-directed violence."[1] The objective of this project was to assist the Air Force in identifying approaches for expanding the Air Force's TFTN program, including estimating each approach's associated manpower requirements, recruiting requirements, total costs, and implementation timelines. Our goal was not to assess the effectiveness of the embedded program model or of the program itself, but rather to develop a model to project provider staffing and program costs based on three potential courses of action.

The research reported here was originally commissioned by Brig Gen Michael E. Martin, Director of Air Force Resilience (AF/A1Z), and conducted within the Manpower, Personnel, and Training Program of RAND Project AIR FORCE from August 2018 to May 2019 as part of a project titled "Alternative Approaches for Expanding Task Force True North."

RAND Project AIR FORCE

RAND Project AIR FORCE (PAF), a division of the RAND Corporation, is the Department of the Air Force's (DAF's) federally funded research and development center for studies and analyses, supporting both the United States Air Force and the United States Space Force. PAF provides the DAF with independent analyses of policy alternatives affecting the development, employment, combat readiness, and support of current and future air, space, and cyber forces. Research is conducted in four programs: Strategy and Doctrine; Force Modernization and Employment; Resource Management; and Workforce, Development, and Health. The research reported here was prepared under contract FA7014-16-D-1000.

Additional information about PAF is available on our website:
www.rand.org/paf/

This report documents work originally shared with the DAF incrementally in several briefings during late 2018 and early 2019. The draft report, issued on May 29, 2019, was reviewed by formal peer reviewers and DAF subject-matter experts.

---

[1] U.S. Air Force, *Task Force-True North Charter*, December 21, 2016.

Acknowledgments

The authors would like to extend thanks to our U.S. Air Force sponsor, who provided valuable feedback on various briefings over the course of this study. In particular, we would like to thank Brig Gen Michael E. Martin. We are also grateful to our action officer, Col Mark Ramsey, who was very helpful in providing oversight of this research effort.

We also note that we could not have completed this work without the support of the Task Force True North team in the Air Force Directorate of Integrated Resilience. In addition, we appreciate the perspectives from individuals from the other services who provided us information on how they manage their embedded health care provider programs. We are grateful for their assistance with our efforts to collect information for this study.

Finally, we also benefited from the contributions of our RAND colleagues, including Ray Conley and Kirsten Keller, who provided incredibly helpful feedback on this report, as well as our peer reviewers, Sarah Meadows and Brittany Clayton, and the RAND Project AIR FORCE quality assurance team, led by David Orletsky.

We retain full responsibility for the objectivity, accuracy, and analytic integrity of the work presented here.

Summary

The Air Force aims to maximize airman fitness and minimize threats to individual and unit readiness. Negative outcomes, such as domestic and sexual violence and suicide, and their associated effects on readiness, can be avoided by increasing airman fitness and ensuring that effective prevention and treatment programs reach those in need. It is this premise that drives the Air Force's Task Force True North (TFTN) program, which makes the assumption that the Air Force can prevent these behavioral threats to readiness by increasing access to health services by embedding health care providers directly into units. We did not evaluate this assumption in this project.

The objective of this project was to assist the Air Force in identifying approaches to expanding its TFTN program, including estimating each approach's associated manpower requirements, recruiting requirements, total costs, and implementation timelines. Our goal was not to assess the effectiveness of the embedded program model or of the TFTN program itself, but rather to develop a model to project provider staffing and program costs based on three potential courses of action for program expansion.

TFTN was modeled after U.S. Special Operations Command's (USSOCOM's) Preservation of the Force and Family (POTFF) initiative[2] and the Air Force Comprehensive Airman Fitness (CAF) framework, which is described in Air Force Instruction (AFI) 90-5001.[3] The CAF

> is a holistic, strength-based, and integrated framework that plays a role in sustaining a fit, resilient, and ready force. It includes fitness in the mental, physical, social, and spiritual domains, and incorporates the Wingman concept of Airmen taking care of Airmen. CAF is not a standalone program, but encompasses multiagency programs and activities across the Air Force.[4]

Table S.1 shows the CAF fitness "domains," with the analogous POTFF performance areas below them in parentheses. The second column of the table shows the tenets of the Air Force domain. The third column lists the goals of the analogous POTFF performance area.

---

[2] According to the USSOCOM website, the POTFF mission is "To identify and implement innovative, valuable solutions across the USSOCOM Enterprise aimed at improving the short and long-term well-being of our SOF warriors and their families" (USSOCOM, undated). The initial POTFF contract was awarded in January 2013 (Koufas, 2016).

[3] AFI 90-5001, 2019. Also see Robinson, 2019a.

[4] AFI 90-5001, 2019, paragraph 1.3.

Table S.1. Comprehensive Airman Fitness Domains and Tenets with POTFF Analogues

Fitness Domain (POTFF Performance Area)	Air Force Domain Tenets	POTFF Performance Area
Mental (psychological performance)	Awareness – Adaptability – Decision Making – Positive Thinking	• Designed to improve the cognitive and behavioral performance of the force. • Includes helping service members cope with stress, building upon existing strengths, to improve the readiness of special operations forces (SOF) and their families
Physical (human performance)	Endurance – Recovery – Nutrition – Strength	• Meet the unique physical needs of SOF operators with holistic, embedded treatment and training • Maintain operators' peak performance throughout their 20–30-year careers
Social (social and family performance)	Communication – Connectedness – Social Support – Teamwork	• Incorporates family resilience programs designed to enhance service-provided programs • Programs are adapted for the uniqueness of the SOF family
Spiritual (spiritual performance)	Core Values – Perseverance – Perspective – Purpose	• Designed to enhance core spiritual beliefs, values, awareness, relationships, and experiences

SOURCES: AFI 90-5001, 2019, Table 1.1; USSOCOM website (USSOCOM, 2019).

The Military's Rationale for Embedded Care

The military's rationale for relying on embedded care providers is that stigma associated with seeking mental health care, as well as other perceived barriers to care, can be circumvented by bringing the care directly to the service member. In addition to *proximity*, embedding providers can increase the *continuity* of care delivered to service members throughout a deployment cycle. There is also a commonly held belief that providers assigned to units will reduce *stigma* associated with seeking care by forging relationships with unit members and understanding their experiences and culture, thus establishing more provider "credibility." Stigma may also be reduced by demonstrating to service members that their command and senior leaders are supportive of behavioral health care. Embedded providers can also benefit commanders by providing a single point of contact for understanding mental fitness–related concerns and an opportunity to build *trust* with the provider. The embedded providers' presence alone may raise mental health awareness in commanders and service members. Embedded providers are also well positioned to recognize problems in service members before they become severe enough to require referral to specialty health care. Early recognition and early intervention can prevent threats to unit readiness and tragic outcomes. We did not conduct a systematic or in-depth review of the literature on embedded care to test these assumptions. Rather, we began with the assumption the Air Force makes: that embedding care can improve the health of the force.

Examples of Embedded Provider Programs from the Other Military Services

Each of the other services in the U.S. military has experience with embedded behavioral or physical health programs, though the structure, focus, and results of each vary. While some studies that have been conducted point to advantages of certain embedded program designs, overall, the research is limited, and a systematic literature review of embedded care was beyond the scope of the current study. But it is clear from the interviews with leaders of embedded programs that benefits and drawbacks result from each type of embedded care model. Because of the diversity in program design and implementation across the services, each program offers opportunities to draw lessons learned for the Air Force's expansion of TFTN. In addition, USSOCOM has substantial experience in developing and implementing an embedded health program throughout its units and special operations components in each of the services.

Although not exhaustive, our analysis of the interviews with leaders of the embedded health programs in the Army, Navy, Marine Corps, and USSOCOM shows that each service administers its program in ways substantially different than the others. For example, the degree of standardization among the programs ranges from very little, as is the case with USSOCOM's POTFF initiative, to highly standardized, as in the Army's Embedded Behavioral Health (EBH) program. Further, organizational structure, chain of command, and the personnel included in provider teams also varies widely among the other services and USSOCOM. Each program has its own strengths and trade-offs and can offer critical lessons for the Air Force's efforts.

Despite variations in program design and implementation, through interviews with program stakeholders, we identified some key commonalities that characterize the other services' and USSOCOM's programs:

- First and foremost, program design must follow directly from program goals, rather than the inverse. The type of specific program goal of the embedded program—for example, to increase readiness, to provide better medical care for the service member, to strengthen relationships between providers and units—will directly affect how the program should be structured, whether providers should fall within the unit chain of command, and how data on program effectiveness should be collected.
- Second, all embedded providers need to be able to build trust and buy-in with both unit commanders and service members. Interviewees we spoke with emphasized two key elements in forging those relationships: (1) effective training in and/or underlying understanding of specific unit needs and unit and service culture and (2) actual embedding within the units to increase repeat interaction, increase accessibility, and normalize treatment so that stigma is lessened. Further, each interviewee stressed that providers need to understand the unit's responsibilities and unique characteristics in order to be able to correctly determine whether a service member is fit for duty.
- Third, even if programs are not centralized or standardized across all units, data collection should be centralized so that the service can better disseminate lessons learned, have adequate information to effectively advocate for additional resources, and better

target efforts to address program goals, whether in specific units or across the service's program.

RAND Framework for Squadron Risk Levels and Personnel Packages

During the course of this study, we developed a framework for analyzing mental, physical, and social squadron risk levels. To identify where squadron manpower needs may be greater, we first sought to identify the squadrons that might be at highest risk, as well as a method for assessing risk that the Air Force could use in the future. Our squadron risk framework and our initial assessment of squadron risk served as a foundation for the Air Force TFTN team's further assessments of risk. The TFTN team was able to access additional data sources suggested by RAND related to sensitive topics, such as sexual assault, suicide, and problematic behaviors, which allowed the Air Force to build an even more robust data set on risk metrics. We recommend that the Air Force continue to build on the risk framework and risk assessment developed by RAND and continue to acquire additional data to inform its evolving risk metrics. The next section describes our risk framework and its risk assessment.

Unit Risk and Protective Factors

Looking at the common risk factors across negative outcomes is useful for developing efficient support services. In a 2017 study, RAND researchers reviewed risk factors for sexual harassment, sexual assault, unlawful discrimination, substance abuse, suicide, and hazing, seeking to identify risk factors that were common across those problematic behaviors. They found substantial empirical evidence that climate is associated with sexual assault, sexual harassment, unlawful discrimination, substance abuse, and suicide.[5] Prior engagement in the problematic behavior, attitudes toward it, and access to means all increase the likelihood of these problematic behaviors. In an earlier study, the researchers also reviewed research on prevention strategies and found that education, skills building and social support, bystander support, and changes to attitudes, norms, and culture are viable prevention strategies.[6] Embedded providers may be well positioned to offer these prevention services to their units.

Data and Metrics Used for Independent RAND Risk Framework and Assessment

The first step that we took in determining a squadron's risk and its degree of need for assistance in any of the CAF domains was to establish some measures of the current status of each domain. To do so, we made use of data and approaches developed by the Air Force's 711th Human Performance Wing at the Air Force Research Laboratory (AFRL/711th HPW), detailed data from the Air Force's Military Personnel Data System (MilPDS), and analyses from earlier

---

[5] Marquis et al., 2017.

[6] Marquis et al., 2017.

RAND research. These data sources enabled us to develop risk metrics for the physical, mental, and social domains. Because of the lack of available data, we were unable to develop any metrics for the spiritual domain. Table S.2 shows how our variables were combined to determine squadron risk levels in the physical, mental, and social domains.

Table S.2. Variables Used to Determine Risk Levels in Each Domain

Domain	Risk Determination
Physical	Average of the unit percentile for the MilPDS "non-deployable for physical reasons" variable and the unit percentile for musculoskeletal injury risk factor
Mental	Average of the unit percentile for mental health risk factor and the unit percentile for suicide risk factor
Social	Average of the unit percentile for the MilPDS social detractor variable,[a] installation-level risk for female sexual assault, and installation-level risk for male sexual assault

[a] The "social detractor" variable shows the percentage of military personnel in a squadron who had any of the following social risk factors in the past five years: Article 15, court martial, date of earliest return from overseas denied for cause, demotion or withheld promotion, drugs (conviction or in rehabilitation).

After ranking squadrons in each domain, we categorized them as being at high, medium, or low risk in each domain, as follows:

- High risk: top 5 percent of squadrons by risk
- Medium risk: the next 10 percent of squadrons
- Low risk: the remaining 85 percent of squadrons.

Analysis of Personnel Package Composition

We are not aware of any data on the relative effectiveness of one type of embedded provider versus another. Therefore, we looked to the types of providers that are currently included in other examples of embedded provider programs. We strongly recommend that, as the Air Force expands the TFTN program, it carefully track the effectiveness of the different types of providers included in the packages. In particular, if there is variation across the composition of the personnel packages, it is especially important to capture the difference in outcomes across those personnel packages.

Drawing on examples from other embedded provider programs and after discussions with our sponsor, we developed the personnel packages for low-, medium-, and high-risk squadrons shown in Table S.3.

Table S.3. Personnel Packages for Low-, Medium-, and High-Risk Squadrons

Personnel Category	Mental			Social			Physical		
	Low	Medium	High	Low	Medium	High	Low	Medium	High
Licensed clinical social worker	X	X	X		X	X			
Clinical psychologist			X			X			
Mental health technician	X	X	X						
Community support coordinator				X	X	X			
Physical therapist								X	X
Strength and conditioning coach									X
Performance nutritionist									X
Exercise physiologist									X

With the composition of personnel packages defined for the different risk levels by CAF domain, the categorization of the risk levels of each squadron allowed us to estimate the costs of providing these packages to squadrons that need them.

FY 2020–2025 Cost Summary

Table S.4 summarizes the costs of our independent analysis of squadron risk and personnel packages from fiscal years (FYs) 2020 to 2025. The phasing assumptions of the costs come from an initial Program Objective Memorandum (POM) estimate completed by the Air Force for TFTN. Costs are shown by risk domain (social, physical, and mental) and military and civilian personnel.

Table S.4. Full Cost of Manpower Military Cost Categories

Personnel Type	Risk Domain	FY 2020	FY 2021	FY 2022	FY 2023	FY 2024	FY 2025
Military	Social	$0	$105	$197	$226	$246	$251
	Physical	$0	$288	$537	$617	$671	$686
	Mental	$0	$231	$431	$495	$539	$550
Civilian	Social	$0	$6	$10	$12	$13	$13
	Physical	$0	$0	$0	$0	$0	$0
	Mental	$0	$5	$10	$12	$13	$13
Total		**$0**	**$635**	**$1,185**	**$1,361**	**$1,482**	**$1,513**

NOTES: All costs are in millions of then year dollars. Some numbers may not sum correctly because of rounding.

Summary of Alternative Courses of Action and Estimating the Cost of Providing TFTN Personnel Packages

Four alternatives or courses of action (COAs) were developed in collaboration with the Air Force TFTN team:

- Baseline: TFTN POM submission with four-year implementation period
- COA 1: modified POM submission assumptions with five-year implementation period
- COA 2: COA 1 assumptions with ten-year implementation period
- COA 3: five-year implementation with personnel reductions in physical health.

We refer to the first COA simply as the baseline. This COA was the initial Air Force position and is based on the assumptions included in the Air Force–developed FY 2021 POM submission. The personnel packages for each mental health and physical health risk level are summarized in Tables S.5 and S.6. There are four risk levels, ranging from "high+" to "low."[7] The Air Force evaluated each unit type for a risk level and assigned a personnel package based on the identified risk level.[8] As shown in the second column, personnel are embedded at either the squadron level or the group level, providing services to multiple squadrons. Generally speaking, the higher risk the unit type, the more resources embedded at the squadron level.

COA 1: Modified POM Submission with Five-Year Implementation

COA 1 includes the first set of adjustments the Air Force made to the baseline POM estimate. The three major changes are the addition of one year to the implementation schedule, changes to several unit type risk characterizations for both mental health and physical health, and changes in year of implementation for several of the unit types.

COA 2: Ten-Year Implementation

COA 2 includes most of the same assumptions from COA 1 but extends the implementation to ten years in an attempt to reduce the five-year Future Years Defense Program (FYDP) cost by slowing the ramp-up.

COA 3: Five-Year Implementation with Reductions in Physical Health Personnel

COA 3 returns to the COA 1 implementation schedule of five years. The major change in this COA is the reduction in physical health personnel. All maintenance and logistics readiness–related squadrons are assumed to receive their respective squadron-level personnel packages at the group level rather than embedded at each individual squadron.

---

[7] High+ squadrons are those squadrons that the Air Force has prioritized for TFTN resources.

[8] The basic unit in the Air Force is the squadron. Three or more squadrons typically form a group.

Table S.5. Mental Health Personnel Packages, by Risk Level

Mental Health Unit Risk Level	Implementation Level	Job Title
High+	Group	Clinical Psychologist
High+	Group	Mental Health Technician
High+	Squadron	Clinical Psychologist
High	Group	Clinical Psychologist
High	Group	Mental Health Technician
High	Squadron	LCSW[a]
Medium	Group	Mental Health Technician
Medium	Squadron	LCSW[a]
Low	Group	Mental Health Technician
Low	Group	LCSW

[a] LCSW = licensed clinical social worker. For squadrons identified as 24-hour operations, an additional LCSW is included for full coverage. This includes aircraft maintenance, missile maintenance, security forces, missile security, logistics readiness, and intelligence squadrons.

Table S.6. Physical Health Personnel Packages, by Risk Level

Physical Health Unit Risk Level	Implementation Level	Job Title
High+	Group	Performance Nutritionist
High+	Squadron	Exercise Physiologist
High+	Squadron	Strength and Conditioning Coach
High+	Squadron	Physical Therapist
High+	Squadron	Nutritional Medicine Technician
High	Group	Performance Nutritionist
High	Squadron	Exercise Physiologist
High	Squadron	Strength and Conditioning Coach
High	Squadron	Physical Therapist
Medium	Group	Physical Therapist

Comparison of COAs

Table S.7 compares the annual cost based on the cumulative addition of personnel for each of the four alternatives described above. Unsurprisingly, the least expensive option at year 10 is COA 3, because it is the only COA under which personnel are actually reduced. The other three alternatives are relatively close in cost at year 10. At year 5, which would encompass the initial FYDP or budgetary period, the least expensive option is COA 2. This is because the implementation is much slower over a ten-year period.

Table S.7. Comparison of COA Cost Estimates

	Year 1 FY 2021	Year 2 FY 2022	Year 3 FY 2023	Year 4 FY 2024	Year 5 FY 2025	Year 6 FY 2026	Year 7 FY 2027	Year 8 FY 2028	Year 9 FY 2029	Year 10 FY 2030
Baseline	$302	$482	$517	$590	$612	$636	$661	$686	$712	$738
COA 1	$244	$344	$542	$578	$649	$673	$699	$725	$751	$779
COA 2	$170	$259	$362	$450	$509	$609	$643	$673	$725	$779
COA 3	$225	$281	$476	$511	$581	$604	$628	$652	$677	$703

NOTES: All costs are in millions of TY dollars. Some numbers may not sum correctly because of rounding. All cost estimates include 60 religious personnel added annually through year 10.

Monitoring the Expansion of Task Force True North

Monitoring something as sensitive and significant as service member fitness and readiness requires constant vigilance from Air Force leadership and the institution itself. It is not enough to conduct yearly reviews of personnel policies or collect data or statistics. A monitoring plan must consist of long-term and deliberate methods of measuring progress and must include strategies to measure institutional and cultural change over time. A sample monitoring plan is included in Chapter 6.

Establishing and maintaining a monitoring framework is a necessary condition to secure the success of TFTN. Long-term, sustained routine monitoring can identify potential problems quickly as they evolve over time. But the monitoring framework alone is not sufficient for sustained success of TFTN. We recommend that the Air Force also periodically conduct a comprehensive evaluation of the integration process to reevaluate monitoring priorities. A rigorous evaluation that uses valid and reliable research methods can give the Air Force a formal assessment of the process and outcomes of TFTN. We recommend that an initial evaluation be conducted about three years after implementation and then every five years.

Recommendations

The planning phase presents the Air Force with a critical window of opportunity to develop strategies, plans, and policies, as well as to put the necessary data systems in place to monitor the expansion of TFTN over time. Insights from other services' experiences with embedded provider programs and the literature on organizational change inform the following recommendations:[9]

---

[9] See Kotter (1990), Moran and Brightman (2000), Beckhard and Harris (1987), Van De Ven and Poole (1995), and Cummings and Worley (1993).

- Ensure top leadership support and commitment.
- Clarify program goals to enable success.
- Plan up front to facilitate data collection and evaluation.
- Consider issues of chain of command and organizational structure.
- Be prepared to respond to changing needs.
- Monitor progress of implementation over time.

During this planning process, both near-term and long-term issues should be considered, and the mechanisms put into place during the planning process should be flexible enough to accommodate learning and adjustments. Program implementation will likely be a process of continual, iterative improvements. Putting the systems in place to collect the appropriate data throughout the implementation process will help to build the evidence base for those improvements along the way and will facilitate program success.

Contents

About This Report iii

Summary v

Tables xvii

Chapter 1. Introduction 1

    Background and Study Purpose 1

    Study Approach 4

    Caveats and Limitations 5

    Organization of This Report 5

Chapter 2. Maintaining Fitness and Managing Risk Using Embedded Healthcare 7

    Fitness and Readiness 7

    Maintaining Comprehensive Airman Fitness 8

    Unit Risk and Protective Factors 15

    Defining Embedded Care 15

    The Military's Rationale for Embedded Care 16

Chapter 3. Examples of Embedded Health Provider Programs in the Other Military Services 18

    Overview 18

    Army (Embedded Behavioral Health) 19

    Navy (Embedded Mental Health) 23

    U.S. Marine Corps (Operational Stress Control and Readiness) 28

    U.S. Special Operations Command (Preservation of the Force and Family) 33

    Conclusion 37

Chapter 4. RAND Framework for Squadron Risks, Development of Personnel Packages, and

    Assessments of Costs 38

    RAND Framework and Assessment of Squadron Risk Factors 38

    Analysis of Personnel Package Composition 42

    Estimate of Initial TFTN Personnel Packages 44

    Cost of RAND's Initial Independent Assessment of Providing TFTN Personnel Packages 44

    Conclusion 47

Chapter 5. Alternative Courses of Action for Expanding TFTN 48

    The Air Force's Risk Framework and Personnel Packages 48

    Summary of Alternative Courses of Action for Expanding TFTN 50

    Baseline: TFTN POM Submission with Four-Year Implementation Period 50

    COA 1: Modified POM Submission with Five-Year Implementation 55

    COA 2: Ten-Year Implementation 57

    COA 3: Five-Year Implementation with Reductions in Physical Health Personnel 59

    Comparison of COAs 62

Chapter 6. Monitoring the Expansion of Task Force True North 64
    Our Approach to a Monitoring Framework 64
    The Need for Evaluation 67
    Conclusion 67
Chapter 7. Recommendations 68
    Ensure Top Leadership Support and Commitment 68
    Clarify Program Goals to Enable Success 68
    Plan Up Front to Facilitate Data Collection and Evaluation 69
    Consider Issues of Chain of Command and Organizational Structure 69
    Be Prepared to Respond to Changing Needs 70
    Monitor Progress of Implementation over Time 70
    Closing Thoughts 70

Appendix A. Air Force Research Laboratory Profile Risk Score Methodology 71
Appendix B. Semistructured Interview Protocol 72
Abbreviations 73
References 75

Tables

Table S.1. Comprehensive Airman Fitness Domains and Tenets with POTFF Analogues vi

Table S.2. Variables Used to Determine Risk Levels in Each Domain ix

Table S.3. Personnel Packages for Low-, Medium-, and High-Risk Squadrons.........................x

Table S.4. Full Cost of Manpower Military Cost Categories................................x

Table S.5. Mental Health Personnel Packages, by Risk Level.........................xii

Table S.6. Physical Health Personnel Packages, by Risk Level xii

Table S.7. Comparison of COA Cost Estimates..........................xiii

Table 1.1. Comprehensive Airman Fitness Domains and Tenets with POTFF Analogues 4

Table 4.1. MilPDS Indicators of Risk in the Physical and Social Domains 40

Table 4.2. Data Sources and Applicable CAF Domains 41

Table 4.3. Variables Used to Determine Initial Risk Levels in Each Domain........................42

Table 4.4. Comparison of POTFF, OST, and TFTN Test Program Personnel Packages 43

Table 4.5. Personnel Packages for Low-, Medium-, and High-Risk Squadrons.........................44

Table 4.6. Full Cost of Manpower Military Cost Categories........................45

Table 4.7. Full Cost of Manpower Government Civilian Cost Categories 46

Table 4.8. Cost Estimate Summary 47

Table 5.1. Air Force Mental Health Personnel Packages, by Risk Level.........................49

Table 5.2. Air Force Physical Health Personnel Packages, by Risk Level 49

Table 5.3. Personnel Type and Pay Grade Assumptions for COA Cost Estimates.........................52

Table 5.4. Baseline Mental Health and Physical Health Unit Risk Summary 53

Table 5.5. Baseline Cost Estimate..........................54

Table 5.6. Baseline Personnel Count..........................54

Table 5.7. COA 1 Mental Health and Physical Health Unit Risk Summary.........................55

Table 5.8. COA 1 Cost Estimate 56

Table 5.9. COA 1 Personnel Count 57

Table 5.10. COA 2 Mental Health and Physical Health Unit Risk Summary.........................57

Table 5.11. COA 2 Cost Estimate 59

Table 5.12. COA 2 Personnel Count..........................59

Table 5.13. COA 3 Mental Health and Physical Health Unit Risk Summary.........................60

Table 5.14. COA 3 Cost Estimate 61

Table 5.15. COA 3 Personnel Count 62

Table 5.16. Comparison of COA Cost Estimates..........................62

Table 6.1. Sample Framework for Monitoring the Expansion of TFTN.........................65

Chapter 1. Introduction

Background and Study Purpose

The Air Force aims to maximize airman fitness and minimize threats to individual and unit readiness. Negative outcomes, such as domestic and sexual violence and suicide, can be avoided by increasing airman fitness and by ensuring that effective prevention and treatment programs reach those in need. It is this premise that drives the Air Force's Task Force True North (TFTN) program. The assumption is that the Air Force can prevent these behavioral threats to readiness by increasing access to health services by embedding health care providers directly into units.

After the wars in Iraq and Afghanistan began, concerns about the psychological impacts of deployments led to the development of pre-deployment preparation, forward-deployed combat stress support teams, and post-deployment reintegration programs. In 2002, the *New York Times* reported on a string of murder-suicides involving three recently returned war veterans.[10] This raised awareness of the impacts of war on service members.

The extent of mental health symptoms plaguing service members who deployed to Iraq became clearer with the first publication of the Walter Reed Army Institute of Research's Land Combat Study.[11] The authors detailed rates of positive screening for depression and posttraumatic stress disorder (PTSD) and described a problematic pattern—those with the most significant mental health challenges perceived greater stigma associated with seeking treatment than did those without mental health symptoms.[12] Evidence of mental health stigma as a barrier to seeking mental health care and congressional and public concern about the military's capacity to deliver high-quality mental health care to all who needed it led to significant changes in the way care is delivered. Embedding providers represented a significant shift in the military health care delivery model.

President George W. Bush issued Executive Order 13426, *Establishing a Commission on Care for America's Returning Wounded Warriors and a Task Force on Returning Global War on Terror Heroes*, on March 6, 2007. The charge for the resulting "Dole-Shalala Commission" was "to provide a comprehensive review of the care provided to America's returning Global War on Terror service men and women from the time they leave the battlefield through their return to civilian life."[13] In July 2007, the commission published 95 recommendations on how to improve the psychological health of service members and their families.

---

[10] Associated Press, 2002.

[11] Hoge et al., 2004.

[12] Hoge et al., 2004; Hoge, Auchterlonie, and Milliken, 2006.

[13] President's Commission on Care for America's Returning Wounded Warriors, 2007.

One of the U.S. Department of Defense's (DoD)'s responses to the commission's recommendations was to embed behavioral health (BH) providers in theaters of war.[14] The 2007 *DoD Plan to Achieve the Vision of the DoD Task Force on Mental Health* stated that to build psychological fitness and resilience while dispelling stigma, DoD would embed operational psychological health providers in line units to be "trusted advisors to line leaders and trusted supporters of our military Service members."[15] DoD planned to rely on existing models, such as the Operational Stress Control and Readiness (OSCAR) program in the Marine Corps and the embedded providers in special operations forces (SOF) units in the Army and Air Force, to form a core set of principles to deploy across DoD (see Chapter 3 for additional detail on these programs). DoD planned to then pilot core programs to refine the processes and training and create career paths for embedded providers.[16]

Medical support teams have always existed in theaters of war, but this new model of embedded care places the providers in the units themselves. Moving beyond the health care setting, embedding mental health providers in units was expected to decrease mental health stigma by showing service members that command supports mental health care and by inculcating providers into unit culture, so that service members might have more trust in the provider.

With increased attention to service member mental health came money for DoD to implement new procedures for managing mental health problems. A mass of epidemiologic research on the risk factors associated with development of psychological problems grew, and programs designed to help service members and their families proliferated—so much so that a 2011 RAND study documented 211 programs to support psychological health and traumatic brain injuries in service members and families.[17] This created a difficult-to-navigate system of support, and evaluations of services were scarce, which meant the effectiveness of these care models in military populations was largely unknown.[18]

TFTN was modeled after U.S. Special Operations Command's (USSOCOM's) Preservation of the Force and Family (POTFF) initiative[19] and the Air Force Comprehensive Airman Fitness (CAF) framework, which is described in Air Force Instruction (AFI) 90-5001.[20] The CAF

---

[14] DoD, 2007.

[15] DoD, 2007, p. 5.

[16] DoD, 2007, p. 5.

[17] Weinick et al., 2011.

[18] Institute of Medicine, 2014; Engel et al., 2008.

[19] According to the USSOCOM website, the POTFF mission is "To identify and implement innovative, valuable solutions across the USSOCOM Enterprise aimed at improving the short and long-term well-being of our SOF warriors and their families" (USSSCOM, undated). The initial POTFF contract was awarded in January 2013 (Koufas, 2016).

[20] AFI 90-5001, 2019. See also Robinson, 2019a.

... is a holistic, strength-based, and integrated framework that plays a role in sustaining a fit, resilient, and ready force. It includes fitness in the mental, physical, social, and spiritual domains, and incorporates the Wingman concept of Airmen taking care of Airmen. CAF is not a standalone program, but encompasses multiagency programs and activities across the Air Force. It is a cultural shift in how we view and maintain fitness in a more comprehensive manner and enables Airmen to hold each other accountable against Air Force Core Values. Leaders and individuals throughout the Total Force are to understand, support, and promote the CAF framework.[21]

Table 1.1 shows the CAF fitness "domains," with the analogous POTFF performance areas below them in parentheses. The second column of the table shows the tenets of the Air Force domain. The third column lists the goals of the analogous POTFF performance area.

The CAF defines resilience as "the ability to withstand, recover, and grow in the face of stressors and changing demands."[22] Thus, all CAF pillars are necessary for maintaining resilience.

The objective of this project was to assist the Air Force in identifying approaches to expanding its TFTN program, including estimating each approach's associated manpower requirements, recruiting requirements, total costs, and implementation timelines. Our goal was not to assess the effectiveness of the embedded program model or of the TFTN program itself, but rather to develop a model to project provider staffing and program costs based on three potential courses of action for program expansion.

---

[21] AFI 90-5001, 2019, paragraph 1.3.

[22] AFI 90-5001, 2019, paragraph 1.1.

Table 1.1. Comprehensive Airman Fitness Domains and Tenets with POTFF Analogues

Fitness Domain (POTFF Performance Area)	Air Force Domain Tenets	POTFF Performance Area
Mental (psychological performance)	Awareness – Adaptability – Decision Making – Positive Thinking	• Designed to improve the cognitive and behavioral performance of the force • Includes helping service members cope with stress, building upon existing strengths, to improve the readiness of SOF and their families
Physical (human performance)	Endurance – Recovery – Nutrition – Strength	• Meet the unique physical needs of SOF operators with holistic, embedded treatment and training • Maintain operators' peak performance throughout their 20–30-year careers
Social (social and family performance)	Communication – Connectedness – Social Support – Teamwork	• Incorporates family resilience programs designed to enhance service-provided programs • Programs are adapted for the uniqueness of the SOF family
Spiritual (spiritual performance)	Core Values – Perseverance – Perspective – Purpose	• Designed to enhance core spiritual beliefs, values, awareness, relationships, and experiences

SOURCES: AFI 90-5001, 2019, Table 1.1; USSOCOM website (USSOCOM, 2019).

Study Approach

This study consisted of six tasks: (1) review policy documents and data on the effectiveness of embedded health care in the military services, (2) identify the needs of units and populations that are at high, medium, and low risk for decreased resilience and increased negative outcomes, (3) develop a range of support personnel packages that could be embedded in units that are at high, medium, and low risk for decreased resilience and increased negative outcomes, (4) develop a range of alternative options to expand TFTN, (5) provide a comparative analysis of alternative options to expand TFTN, and (6) document findings and recommendations.

Task 1 consisted of a broad review of the literature on embedded health care programs in the military. We also conducted interviews with subject-matter experts associated with embedded health care programs in the other services. We identified the history, structure, and current implementation of each program in the other DoD services and USSOCOM, and in this report we summarize key points and potential lessons that could be drawn from each.

In Task 2, we independently identified the needs of units and populations that are at high, medium, and low risk for mental, physical, and social fitness. We first established some measures of the current status of each domain. To do so, we made use of data and approaches developed by the Air Force's 711th Human Performance Wing at the Air Force Research Laboratory (AFRL/711th HPW), detailed data from the Air Force's Military Personnel Data System (MilPDS), and analyses from earlier RAND research. These data sources enabled us to develop independent risk metrics for the physical, mental, and social domains.

In Task 3, we independently developed an initial set of TFTN personnel packages for the Air Force. We were not able to find any data on the relative effectiveness of one type of embedded provider versus another; therefore, we looked to the types of providers that are currently included in other examples of embedded provider programs. Using these examples of the types of personnel required for various services and after discussions with our sponsor, we determined the personnel required for low-, medium-, and high-risk squadrons in the three domains.

In Tasks 4 and 5, we worked with our sponsor to develop a range of alternative options for expanding TFTN. We assessed each option against a range of criteria, including costs, implementation timeline, and risks.

In Task 6, we documented the findings from the various analyses conducted during the course of the study, and all the previous tasks fed into the development of a monitoring framework. This monitoring framework offers suggestions for how the Air Force might think about monitoring the expansion of TFTN. Finally, we looked across all of our findings to develop recommendations to the Air Force on how to manage and monitor the expansion of TFTN.

Caveats and Limitations

A critical limitation of our analysis is the lack of rigorous evaluations of embedded health care provider programs in the U.S. military. Much of the existing research on embedded health care provider programs relies on utilization rates of these programs rather than outcomes. As a result, it is important for the Air Force to monitor the expansion of the TFTN program closely and capture lessons learned along the way.

In addition, it is important to note that at the time this study was undertaken, the TFTN program had not been formally evaluated yet, so it was unclear whether the TFTN program was meeting its program goals. The RAND team was not asked to evaluate and provide recommendations on whether the TFTN program should be expanded. Instead, we were charged by the Air Force to assume that the TFTN program would be expanded. Therefore, the question of whether the program should or should not be expanded was beyond the scope of this study.

Organization of This Report

Chapter 2 describes DoD's fitness framework, risk and protective factors for poor fitness, and prevention and treatment approaches. The chapter then discusses the definition of *embedded care* and the rationale for its use. Chapter 3 describes the embedded health programs that each of the services and USSOCOM have implemented and lessons learned from these programs. Chapter 4 presents the framework that we developed to help the Air Force identify mental, physical, and social risk rankings of Air Force squadrons. Chapter 5 presents a summary of costs for four alternatives for expanding the TFTN program. Chapter 6 presents a framework for monitoring the implementation of the expansion of TFTN. Chapter 7 discusses our conclusions and recommendations. Appendix A presents the Air Force Research Laboratory's risk methodology. Appendix B presents our semistructured interview protocol.

Chapter 2. Maintaining Fitness and Managing Risk Using Embedded Healthcare

In this chapter, we describe DoD's fitness framework, risk and protective factors for poor fitness, and prevention and treatment approaches. We then discuss the definition of embedded care and the rationale for its use. In the next chapter, we describe the embedded health programs that each of the services and USSOCOM have implemented and lessons learned from these programs.

Fitness and Readiness

Ultimately, the goal of delivering health care and support to service members is to maintain ready airmen and ready units. Force readiness depends on a multitude of factors, including the well-being of each service member. Individual medical readiness, defined in DoD Instruction (DODI) 6025.19, is essential to force readiness. The instruction states that, "service members have a responsibility to maintain their health and fitness, meet individual medical readiness requirements, and report medical (including mental health) and health issues that may affect their readiness to deploy or fitness to continue serving in an active status."[23] To help define individual readiness, DoD created the Total Force Fitness Framework. The purpose of the framework is to "organize the services provided and to educate service members on aspects of individual readiness."[24] The instruction defines eight domains of fitness: physical, environment, medical and dental, nutritional, spiritual, psychological, behavioral, and social.

The Air Force's approach to understanding fitness is called Comprehensive Airman Fitness and is detailed in AFI 90-506. The goal of CAF is to "equip Airmen with tools and skills . . . to maintain a balance of cognitive skills, physical endurance, emotional stamina, and spiritual well-being needed to execute [the] central mission."[25] It defines four fitness domains—mental, physical, social, and spiritual—and states that well-being in these areas is a necessary component of individual readiness. This chapter focuses on maintaining fitness across all four of the CAF domains, as well as unit risk and protective factors and the military's rationale for embedded care.

---

[23] DODI 6025.19, 2014.

[24] Chairman of the Joint Chiefs of Staff Instruction 3405.01, 2011.

[25] AFI 90-506, 2014.

Maintaining Comprehensive Airman Fitness

A vast literature exists on the epidemiology of war-related injuries, risk and protective factors, and prevention and treatment of mental, physical, social, and spiritual issues. Describing the totality of these threats to readiness and best practices for the identification, prevention, and treatment of military health problems is beyond the scope of this report. Nevertheless, understanding specific factors associated with fitness is necessary for determining the prevention and health care resources required to restore and maintain fitness.

The fitness domains are interrelated. Mental fitness affects physical, social, and spiritual fitness and vice versa, so deficits in any domain are a risk factor for other fitness deficits. Thus, prevention efforts may influence all fitness domains, and treatment in one domain may result in increased fitness across domains. For instance, PTSD is associated with military attrition,[26] decreased quality of life,[27] lost workdays,[28] and a host of physical health problems, such as poor sleep, gastro-intestinal disorders, headaches, pain, and cardiovascular outcomes.[29] Treatment can improve all those associated outcomes.

Maintaining Mental Fitness

CAF defines mental fitness as "the ability to effectively cope with unique mental stressors and challenges."[30] Mental fitness problems include psychological adjustment difficulties, PTSD, depression, substance misuse, anxiety, and other psychological disorders.

Risk Factors

Drawing on information from DoD offices responsible for psychological health problem areas, we summarize below the known risk factors for psychological disorders prevalent among members of the military. According to the DoD Psychological Health Center of Excellence (PHCoE), the risk and protective factors for PTSD (before, during, and after the trauma) are[31]

- Pretraumatic factors
    - Childhood adversity
    - Exposure to prior trauma
    - Ongoing life stress
    - Lack of social support
    - Preexisting or family history of psychiatric disorders

---

[26] Hoge, Auchterlonie, and Milliken, 2006.

[27] Schnurr et al., 2009.

[28] Hoge et al., 2007.

[29] Ramchand et al., 2015, p. 37.

[30] AFI 90-506, 2014.

[31] See Psychological Health Center of Excellence (undated-a).

- Young age at time of trauma
- Female gender
- Lower socioeconomic status, lower education, lower intelligence, minority racial/ethnic status

- Peritraumatic factors[32]

  - High perceived life threat
  - Community (mass) trauma
  - Being a perpetrator, witnessing atrocities, or killing the enemy
  - Combat exposure—frequency and intensity of direct exposure
  - Type and magnitude of trauma (with interpersonal traumas, such as torture, rape, or assault associated with higher risk of PTSD)
  - Peritrauma disassociation
  - Severe trauma

- Posttraumatic factors

  - Development of acute stress disorder
  - Ongoing life stress or adverse events
  - Lack of positive social support/negative social support (e.g., negative reactions from others)
  - Bereavement
  - Significant loss of resources.

PHCoE lists the following risk and protective factors associated with suicide-related thoughts and behaviors:[33]

- Chronic risk factors

  - Mental disorders
  - Medical conditions
  - History of a past suicide attempt
  - Financial difficulties
  - Relationship difficulties
  - Legal problems
  - Adverse childhood experiences

- Acute risk factors

  - Loss of employment
  - Loss of a relationship
  - Loss of housing
  - Onset of psychiatric symptoms
  - Loss of status or rank

---

[32] These are factors occurring around the time of the trauma.

[33] Psychological Health Center of Excellence, undated-b.

- Interpersonal assault
- Suicide death of a relative or peer

- Protective factors
  - Employment
  - Responsibilities to others
  - Strong interpersonal bonds
  - Resilience
  - Sense of belonging and identity
  - Access to health care
  - Optimistic outlook.

Other research finds that some mental health problems are risk factors not only for other mental health problems but also for physical fitness, social fitness, and spiritual fitness. For instance, almost half of those with PTSD also have a substance use disorder.[34] And high levels of religiosity and spirituality are associated with decreased risk for PTSD, depression, and alcohol misuse.[35]

Demographic and deployment-related risk factors for PTSD, depression, and substance misuse were reported in a systematic review of primary data collection studies on prevalence, risk factors, and consequences of deployments to Iraq and Afghanistan.[36] The researchers found that (1) women are at greater risk for depression, (2) men are at increased risk for substance misuse, and (3) the relationship between gender and PTSD is complex. Research is equivocal regarding the relationship between gender and post-deployment PTSD.[37] A 2014 meta-analysis of gender differences in post-deployment-related PTSD indicated that it was essential to control for non-deployment-related trauma, as interpersonal trauma is more common in women.[38] Controlling for combat exposure, there appear to be few differences between men and women in the rates of subsequent PTSD; women are more likely to report PTSD from interpersonal trauma, and women who perceive greater betrayal as part of their (interpersonal) trauma have a greater likelihood of developing PTSD.[39]

Research indicates that PTSD is more prevalent among those in health care occupations, combat specialists, and service and supply personnel.[40] Combat exposure is also a stronger

---

[34] Pietrzak et al., 2011.

[35] Sharma et al., 2017.

[36] Ramchand et al., 2015.

[37] Frank et al., 2018.

[38] Crum-Cianflone and Jacobson, 2014.

[39] Frank et al., 2018.

[40] Mayo et al., 2013.

predictor of PTSD than is deployment.[41] Being younger, less educated, lower ranking, and not being in a relationship increase risk for PTSD, depression, and substance misuse.[42]

Prevention and Treatment

Extensive clinical practice guidelines exist for the treatment of acute stress disorder, PTSD, depression, substance misuse, and managing suicide to educate providers about effective interventions.[43] Screening and early recognition of mental health problems can reduce the likelihood of conditions worsening. For instance, one evidence-based early-intervention approach to prevent the worsening of substance misuse is Screening, Brief Interventions, Referral to Treatment (SBIRT).[44] Treatment of acute stress disorder that occurs within one month of trauma exposure can prevent the development of chronic PTSD.[45] Embedded providers may be well positioned for early recognition and early intervention.

Maintaining Physical Fitness

CAF defines physical fitness as "the ability to adopt and sustain healthy behaviors needed to enhance health and well-being."[46] The rationale is that by optimizing physical fitness, injuries will be reduced. The Army Public Health Center has published rates of injuries, risk factors, and prevention strategies and has noted that about half of service members experience one or more injuries each year, resulting in more than 2 million medical encounters annually across the military services. Injuries are typically exercise- and sports-related, including overuse strains, sprains, and stress fractures, mostly to lower extremities (ankle/foot, knee/lower leg); back and shoulder injuries are also frequent and associated with lifting and carrying activities.[47]

The U.S. Department of Health and Human Services' Office of Disease Prevention and Health Promotion relied on an expert committee to develop a set of leading health indicators. Nutrition, physical activity, and obesity are among them. That office establishes the health targets for the U.S. population, "Healthy People 2020."[48] Healthy People 2020 establishes health objectives with ten-year targets to guide national health promotion efforts. The Centers for Disease Control and Prevention regularly administers the National Health and Nutrition Examination Survey to track health trends to influence health policies.

---

[41] Smith et al., 2008.

[42] Ramchand et al., 2015.

[43] U.S. Department of Veterans Affairs (VA) and DoD, 2013, 2015, 2016, 2017.

[44] Agerwala and McCance-Katz, 2012.

[45] American Psychiatric Association, 2013.

[46] AFI 90-506, 2014.

[47] Army Public Health Center, 2018.

[48] U.S. Department of Health and Human Services, Office of Disease Prevention and Health Promotion, 2020.

Risk Factors

Physical health and healthy behaviors are measured with questions about physical activity, weight status, routine medical care, sleep health, sedentary time, texting while driving, risky sexual behavior, and more.[49] All these factors affect physical fitness. The DoD Health Related Behaviors Survey regularly assesses the health behaviors of the active component. The 2015 survey found more than half of airmen respondents reported sleeping less than needed, 63 percent were obese according to body mass index, and approximately one-third of airmen reported being "bothered a lot" by pain in the past 30 days.[50]

Researchers evaluated the impact of demographic variables, injury history, and biopsychosocial behaviors on musculoskeletal injuries and physical movement and capabilities. Over one observation year, the factors most predictive of musculoskeletal injury in Army Rangers were smoking, prior surgery, recurrent prior musculoskeletal injury, limited-duty days in the prior year for musculoskeletal injury, asymmetrical ankle dorsiflexion, pain with Functional Movement Screen clearing tests, and decreased performance on the two-mile run and two-minute sit-up test.[51]

Physical injury itself is associated with increased risk for PTSD and other psychological adjustment challenges.[52] MacGregor and colleagues found that individuals with battle injuries were twice as likely as those with non-battle injuries to screen positive for PTSD. Other predictors of positive PTSD screens were individuals with more serious injuries, those with mental health diagnoses within one year of deployment, and previous battle injuries.[53]

Prevention and Treatment

Strength trainers and physical therapists can help with fitness, injury prevention, and treatment. Air Force public health specialists (Air Force Specialty Code [AFSC] 4E0X1) and officers (43HX) support health promotion and disease prevention efforts. The Army has implemented some programs to help them balance the need for fitness with the need to prevent injuries, such as the U.S. Army Training and Doctrine Command's Baseline Soldier Physical Readiness Requirements and Gender-Neutral Physical Performance Standards, the Master Fitness Trainer program, and the Army Medical Command's Soldier Medical Readiness and Performance Triad Campaigns.[54] Embedded providers could address many of these topics, including weight loss, motivation for exercise, healthy eating, and sleep hygiene.

---

[49] Meadows et al., 2018b.

[50] Meadows et al., 2018a.

[51] Teyhen et al., 2015.

[52] Mayo et al., 2013.

[53] MacGregor et al., 2013.

[54] Nindl et al., 2013.

Maintaining Social Fitness

CAF defines social fitness as "the ability to engage in healthy social networks that promote overall well-being and optimal performance."[55] The Air Force focuses on the "wingman" concept, which emphasizes the care of the person next to you. Air Force doctrine is to provide mutual support to benefit the welfare of fellow wingmen. The CAF instruction mandates two "Wingman Days" per calendar year for activities that focus on supporting one another.

Risk Factors

CAF defines four aspects of social fitness: communication, connectedness, social support, and teamwork. Thus, individuals with poor social skills (communication, conflict resolution) have poorer social fitness. Feelings of connectedness and team cooperation contribute to social fitness, and mental health symptoms can affect levels of social support and the quality of relationships. For instance, one symptom of PTSD is "feeling distant or cutoff from other people."[56] And military factors can contribute to difficulty in relationships. A longitudinal look at administrative data revealed that divorce rates among enlisted service members increased with number of days deployed.[57] Command climate and unit cohesion may also be associated with social fitness, and one's mental health symptoms can affect unit cohesion. Many risk factors for poor social fitness are similar to risk factors for mental fitness. Poor communication, problem-solving, and conflict resolution skills can affect relationship quality and unit cohesion, and deployment stress can affect relationships and social support.

Prevention and Treatment

Preventing social fitness deficits, intervening for early conflict resolution, and other interventions counselors may deliver to help people with mental health problems are viable strategies for maintaining social fitness. Meredith and colleagues defined four aspects of community-level factors associated with psychological resilience: belongingness, cohesion, connectedness, and collective efficacy.[58] These bonds and commitments are important for units, and the more wingmen know one another, the more likely they are to provide support when needed and to prevent tragedy when possible. Embedded providers could help the unit bond, increase healthy communication, and influence command climate.

---

[55] AFI 90-506, 2014.

[56] American Psychiatric Association, 2013.

[57] Negrusa, Negrusa, and Hosek, 2014.

[58] Meredith et al., 2011.

Maintaining Spiritual Fitness

CAF defines spiritual fitness as "the ability to adhere to beliefs, principles, or values needed to persevere and prevail in accomplishing missions," with four components: core values, perseverance, perspective, and purpose.[59] These characteristics also reflect resilience.

Risk Factors

Trauma can shatter one's beliefs about the world, leading one to doubt higher powers, karma, or other beliefs that might offer some sense of order and peace. Perhaps because spirituality is different for everyone, there is a dearth of literature on building spirituality and recovering it after a "loss" of spirituality. Research has found that general spiritual beliefs and anger were associated with poor physical and mental health outcomes in trauma survivors,[60] and that high religiosity and spirituality decreases the risk for mental health problems.[61]

Prevention and Treatment

Military chaplains are an important resource for many reasons, one of which is guaranteed confidentiality, which notably does not exist with military behavioral health providers. There is little research on spiritual fitness relative to mental and physical fitness. In the context of post-deployment reintegration, for example, a systematic literature review identified domains of reintegration and found that spirituality was least represented in the published literature relative to all other domains of post-deployment reintegration.[62]

The U.S. Navy Chaplain Corps developed a guide on spiritual fitness.[63] A 2016 systematic review of research on moral injury, spirituality, and the chaplaincy found 60 articles on the topics, and approximately half of those were positive about the role or potential role that chaplains can play in addressing mental health, trauma, and associated moral injury.[64] A recent systematic review of research on outcomes of chaplain care produced 22 studies, with a conclusion that outcomes research must find a way to respect the integrity of the chaplaincy to produce better outcome measures and research.[65] Another recent study has advocated the use of military chaplains to screen and treat moral injury, producing a guide to helping service members and veterans with moral injuries of war.[66] Embedded chaplains and, to some extent, embedded

---

[59] AFI 90-506, 2014.

[60] Connor, Davidson, and Lee, 2003.

[61] Sharma et al., 2017.

[62] Elnitsky, Fisher, and Blevins, 2017.

[63] See U.S. Navy Chaplain Corps, "Spiritual Fitness Guide," May 2, 2012.

[64] Carey and Hodgson, 2018.

[65] Damen et al., 2020.

[66] Carey and Hodgson, 2018.

mental health providers may be well positioned to support the spiritual fitness needs of their units.

Unit Risk and Protective Factors

Unit risk is not equal to cumulative individual risk of unit members. Unit characteristics such as cohesion, command climate, and shared beliefs and attitudes can influence readiness. A positive command climate is associated with greater psychological resilience among service members,[67] and a poor command climate is associated with a host of problematic outcomes.

Looking at the common risk factors across negative outcomes is useful for developing efficient support services. In a 2017 study, RAND researchers reviewed risk factors for sexual harassment, sexual assault, unlawful discrimination, substance abuse, suicide, and hazing, seeking to identify risk factors that were common across those problematic behaviors. They found substantial empirical evidence that climate is associated with sexual assault, sexual harassment, unlawful discrimination, substance abuse, and suicide.[68] Prior engagement in the problematic behavior, attitudes toward it, and access to means all increase the likelihood of these problematic behaviors. In an earlier study, the authors also reviewed research on prevention strategies and found that education, skills building and social support, bystander support, and changes to attitudes, norms, and culture are viable prevention strategies.[69] Embedded providers may be well positioned to offer these prevention services to their units.

Defining Embedded Care

Different health care models may be characterized as utilizing embedded providers. For the purposes of this report, we consider health care to be *embedded* when the provider is attached with the unit, deploys with the unit, or serves alongside the unit. We distinguish embedded military health care from co-located providers, from integrated care, and from peer support. The roles of embedded providers differ by the setting in which they practice, such as in-theater, in-garrison, or in a clinic. Further, there are "levels" of embeddedness: The provider billet may be attached to the line or to a military treatment facility (MTF); the providers may or may not deploy with the unit; and shared time required by being attached to an MTF means less availability to command and fewer opportunities to build relationships within the unit.

Co-located providers may deliver care at battalion aid stations or MTFs near the service member. For example, the Air Force has long utilized the Behavioral Health Optimization Program, which places (co-locates) a behavioral health provider in the primary care setting for

---

[67] Meredith et al., 2011.

[68] Marquis et al., 2017.

[69] Marquis et al., 2017.

immediate consultations to better integrate care (by increasing communication between primary care and behavioral health providers) and to provide immediate access for patients.

The growing emphasis on peer-to-peer support programs may also be considered an effort to embed additional care in units. A recent systematic review of peer-to-peer support interventions found that peer counseling showed promise in improving physical health outcomes, and peer educators frequently improved social health and engagement.[70] One example of this approach is the Combat Operational Stress Control (COSC) program, which was initially developed by the Marine Corps.[71] This multifaceted approach to stress management and resilience-building trains some line leaders to be master trainers in the unit and requires COSC training for all unit members. This combination of educational programming and embedded access to expert trainers is believed to reinforce the material and demonstrate that senior leaders value individual well-being and care-seeking.

The Military's Rationale for Embedded Care

Early evidence from the Land Combat Study conducted by the Walter Reed Army Institute of Research found that stigma is a barrier to mental health treatment and that only about one-third of those service members who needed treatment sought it.[72] A RAND study by Acosta and colleagues on mental health stigma in the military described stigma as a dynamic construct that occurs within a number of dimensions: oneself, one's social network, one's community, and the general public.[73] Acosta and team detailed existing DoD policies that may perpetuate stigma by characterizing mental health problems in a negative manner. In the past decade, the military has encouraged senior leaders to promote mental health care in a variety of ways to maintain optimal health. For example, the Marine Corps' OSCAR program trains leaders to recognize stress and to support recovery.[74] Besides stigma, perceived barriers to accessing care (locating services, getting appointments, finding time during the workday, and privacy) have also been documented.[75] Mistrust of behavioral health providers is another documented barrier to care.[76] The reality is that health care providers wear two hats: one that serves the patients and one that serves military commanders who need to understand the health and readiness of their service members. That leads to confusion among service members about the extent of confidentiality

---

[70] Ramchand et al., 2017.

[71] Nash, 2006.

[72] Hoge et al., 2004; Hoge, Auchterlonie, and Milliken, 2006.

[73] Acosta et al., 2014.

[74] Nash, 2006.

[75] Hoge, Auchterlonie, and Milliken, 2006; Acosta et al., 2014.

[76] Hoge et al., 2004; Hoge, Auchterlonie, and Milliken, 2006.

protections they will have when seeking behavioral health treatment.[77] For all these reasons and more, assigning or attaching behavioral health providers to the line units became a key solution for increasing utilization of behavioral health care.

The Army deployed more troops to Iraq and Afghanistan than the other services combined.[78] The high operations tempo and some early high-profile tragedies led to efforts to transform the mental health system to capably deliver high-quality, evidence-based health care.[79] The rationale for relying on embedded care providers is that stigma associated with seeking mental health care, as well as other perceived barriers to care, could be circumvented by bringing the care directly to the service member. In addition to *proximity*, embedding providers can increase the *continuity* of care delivered to service members throughout a deployment cycle. There is also a commonly held belief that providers assigned to units will reduce *stigma* associated with seeking care by forging relationships with the units and understanding their experiences and culture, thus establishing more provider "credibility." Stigma may also be reduced by demonstrating to service members that command is supportive of behavioral health care. Embedded providers can also benefit commanders by providing a single point of contact for understanding mental fitness–related concerns and an opportunity to build *trust* with the provider. The providers' presence alone may raise mental health awareness in commanders and service members. Embedded providers are also well positioned to recognize problems in service members before they become severe enough to require referral to specialty health care. Early recognition and early intervention can prevent threats to unit readiness and tragic outcomes.

---

[77] Hoge, Auchterlonie, and Milliken, 2006.

[78] Baiocchi, 2013.

[79] Hoge et al., 2015.

Chapter 3. Examples of Embedded Health Provider Programs in the Other Military Services

Overview

Each of the other services in the U.S. military has experience with embedded behavioral or physical health programs, though the structure, focus, and results of each vary. The Army deployed more troops to Iraq and Afghanistan than the other services combined.[80] The high operations tempo and some early high-profile tragedies led to efforts to transform the mental health system to capably deliver high-quality, evidence-based health care.[81] Some studies point to advantages of certain embedded program designs, but, overall, the research is limited. Nonetheless, it is clear that benefits and drawbacks accrue from each type of model we identified. Because of the diversity in program design and implementation across the services, each program offers opportunities to draw lessons learned for the Air Force's expansion of TFTN. In addition, USSOCOM has substantial experience in developing and implementing an embedded health program throughout its units and special operations components in each of the services.

We conducted interviews with personnel associated with embedded health programs in the Army, Navy, Marine Corps and USSOCOM. Interviewees were identified through program websites and existing relationships with senior leaders in each service. The goal was to interview leaders of embedded health programs in each service and to obtain source documents that guided program implementation. We developed a semistructured interview protocol that we shared prior to each interview (see Appendix B). We conducted six interviews, and in this chapter we describe the contents of each, by service. We did not conduct formal content or thematic analysis. Drawing on those interviews and supporting documentation we analyzed, in this chapter we present the history, structure, and current implementation of each program in the other DoD services and USSOCOM and summarize key points and potential lessons that could be drawn from each.

---

[80] Baiocchi, 2013.

[81] Hoge et al., 2015.

Army (Embedded Behavioral Health)

History

By 2008, the conflicts in Iraq and Afghanistan had resulted in a significant increase in demands for behavioral health care, particularly from soldiers assigned to operational units.[82] In response, Army unit leaders across the nation identified a gap between soldiers who required behavioral health care and the availability of behavioral health care providers. At Fort Carson, Colorado, leaders hypothesized that the gap might have contributed to a high rate of violent incidents there in 2008, when eight homicides were perpetrated by soldiers from units that had experienced heavy combat in theater. Several news outlets, including National Public Radio and the *Washington Post*, ran negative stories regarding behavioral health care at Fort Carson. This prompted several senators and/or their aides to visit the post. Ultimately, an Epidemiologic Consultation (EPICON) was generated, which resulted in several recommendations regarding a model of care, including the idea of embedded behavioral health care:[83]

> The 2nd BCT [brigade combat team] was the first to receive behavioral health support in the embedded model through a complete Army Force Generation cycle. From their redeployment in mid-2009 to deployment in June 2011, the BCT received embedded behavioral health support from a dedicated medical team that provided care from a clinic in the BCT's area of operation.

> Mental health providers were aligned with each battalion, so each battalion commander had a readily accessible behavioral health subject matter expert to evaluate and treat their Soldiers and assist them in optimizing mission readiness and safety.[84]

The Embedded Behavioral Health (EBH) program at Fort Carson did not start as a pilot program, but rather was a local approach to solving a problem.[85] However, based on its success, it was considered a "best practice" program, and the Army expanded it to other locations.[86] After studies by the Massachusetts Institute of Technology (MIT) and Yale University showed the

---

[82] Cho-Stutler, 2013.

[83] Carabajal, 2011; Cho-Stutler, 2013.

[84] Carabajal, 2011.

[85] RAND interview with Army EBH personnel, May 8, 2019.

[86] Carabajal's (2011) article says that

> The program improved access to care, improved continuity of care, enhanced BH provider communication with commanders, decreased inpatient hospitalizations, decreased referrals to the TRICARE network for behavioral health care and garnered high rates of commander and Soldier satisfaction. Additionally, compared to the unit's last deployment before the embedded program was implemented, 2nd BCT had 96 fewer Soldiers left on rear-detachment for a behavioral health reason after receiving a complete cycle of embedded behavioral health support.

effectiveness of these programs,[87] the Army issued Executive Order 236-12 in July 2012, directing "full implementation of EBHTs [embedded behavioral health teams] for all active operational (deployable) units by fiscal year 2016."[88]

Structure of the Army's Embedded Behavioral Health Program

The Army's approach to EBH is described in the *Embedded Behavioral Health Guide*, published by U.S. Army Medical Command in October 2014, with staffing guidelines established in a fragmentary order published in 2015. The commander's intent for EBHT execution is

> to establish multidisciplinary BH teams to improve access to and continuity of behavioral healthcare by moving into closer physical proximity (requirement for Brigade Combat Teams [BCT] only) to Soldiers' work areas, streamlining the number of BH providers involved in the treatment process and forming strong relationships with operational leaders.[89]

According to the *Embedded Behavioral Health Guide*, four core elements guide the structure of EBH:

1. Alignment of behavioral healthcare with the unit being supported (direct support relationships).
2. Continuity by BH personnel throughout the Army Force Generation cycle.
3. Multidisciplinary team-based care centered around the Soldier.
4. Care as close to the point of need as possible (far-forward clinic locations).[90]

The EBH program "converts the MTF's outpatient system of behavior health care from a traditional medical model into a direct support model which aligns multi-disciplinary teams of behavioral health (BH) personnel with specific units."

The Army's structure, which maintains the providers in the MTF's chain of command, as opposed to the embedded unit's chain of command, distinguishes it from other service programs. Program personnel we spoke with felt that this model is both effective and rewarding for several reasons, including that it enables the providers greater ability to speak openly with command leadership about service members' readiness. It also creates space for the command team to

---

[87] RAND interview with Army EBH personnel (May 8, 2019) who provided study materials published through the MIT website: Srinivasan and DeBenigno, 2014; Srinivasan, 2016a, 2016b; DeBenigno, 2016.

[88] *Embedded Behavioral Health Guide* (U.S. Army Medical Command, 2014, p. 5). Executive Order 236-12 (Headquarters, U.S. Army, 2012) was published in July 2012, and U.S. Army Medical Command published Operational Order (OPORD) 12-63 in August 2012, directing MTFs to begin EBH implementation for all deployable units no later than October 2012 and complete it no later than September 2016. Finally, the report of the Army Task Force on Behavioral Health, published in January 2013, includes the recommendation "Expand the Embedded BH program aligning BH providers with brigade level deployable units."

[89] U.S. Army Medical Command, 2015.

[90] U.S. Army Medical Command, 2014, p. 4.

approach the providers for assistance regarding their own personal support, which they might not pursue if the providers were within their chain of command.

Current Implementation and Team Composition

The 2015 fragmentary order for EBHT implementation provides the following guidelines for team composition:[91]

- Behavioral health providers (defined as clinical psychologists and licensed clinical social workers [LCSWs]) will form direct support relationships with specific operational units on the installation. The optimal support ratio is one behavioral health provider per 600–900 soldiers (average one provider per battalion).
- The optimal support ratio for psychology technician and social services assistants is one psychology technician *or* one social services assistant per three behavioral health providers.
- The optimal support ratio for case managers and licensed practical nurses is a ratio of one case manager *and* one licensed practical nurse per EBHT or six behavioral health providers.
- Front desk staff-medical support assistants will be assigned to adequately support the clinical staff (two medical support assistants for stand-alone EBHT).

In addition to these personnel, the brigade behavioral health officer, who is assigned to a U.S. Army Forces Command unit, is considered to be part of the team as borrowed military personnel from the supported brigade.[92]

The EBH clinic serves as the single point of entry into behavioral health care for each battalion soldier and leader, and facilitates early identification and intervention:

> Soldiers receive expedited evaluations and community-level treatment from a single provider, which greatly improves continuity of care. Leaders have a single point of contact for questions regarding the BH of their Soldiers and an easily accessible subject matter expert. The BH provider maintains visibility on the mission readiness and safety status of all assigned Soldiers, identifies trends, and works with line and medical leaders on a regular basis.[93]

An important expectation is that the enduring working relationship between the provider and battalion personnel will erode any stigma that might be associated with behavioral health care in the military setting.

Army EBH providers are assigned to specific units, but they are "owned" by the MTF under the chief of mental health,[94] and their integration into individual units is a matter of *location*. In other words, "EBH integrates BH specialties and aligns them with operational (deployable) units

---

[91] U.S. Army Medical Command, 2015.

[92] U.S. Army Medical Command, 2014, p. 4.

[93] U.S. Army Medical Command, 2014, p. 4.

[94] RAND interview with Army EBH personnel, May 8, 2019.

to deliver outpatient behavioral healthcare to Soldiers in close proximity to their units and optimizes the mission readiness of the force."[95] Also, "locating the EBHT in the physical proximity of a supported unit allows the EBHT to provide multidisciplinary behavioral healthcare to Soldiers in coordination with unit leaders which serves to maximize diagnostic accuracy, reduce barriers to care, and improve treatment outcomes."[96]

The number of people who remain in garrison when a brigade deploys varies, and the EBH team supporting the brigade adjusts its composition and operations according to the needs of the rear-detachment contingent. The brigade behavioral health officer deploys with the unit and is expected to communicate with the EBH team to ensure continuity of care for returning and deployed soldiers. The behavioral health officer is also supposed to be on the first returning flight from a deployment in order to support continuity of care for soldiers.[97]

Key Points and Lessons the Air Force Can Learn from the Army

- **The Army program is, compared with the other services, very highly centralized.** This degree of centralization is by design: It helps to ensure that the program is adopted and employed correctly, and it builds on lessons learned and evidence that the program works. It also provides guidelines for the way interactions between the medical providers and the units should occur, to ensure that the separate, but connected, goals of the medical team and the unit commander are achieved. The program model is not entirely inflexible, but it is distinct from the other services' programs, which are highly dependent on what the commander determines is needed in terms of types of providers and interactions. Centralization also enables the program managers (and Army writ large) to enforce accountability and adoption of the program.

  - Potential Lesson: With clear program goals and evidence of success, centralization can be advantageous, and the Army's model might be more streamlined and effective than a risk-based model.
  - Potential Lesson: Program personalization can be maintained even if the programs are centrally managed with similar designs.

- **Even with centralization and mandated programs, buy-in from unit commanders can be challenging.**

  - Potential Lesson: The service must ensure that commanders and other unit leaders understand the utility of the program, and that providers are equipped to continually reinforce that message.

- **Success of the program is predicated on the foundation that the service must know the program goals and exactly what it wants out of the embedded interactions.** If the program's purpose is not well articulated, outcomes are impossible to measure.

---

[95] U.S. Army Medical Command, 2014, p. 5.

[96] U.S. Army Medical Command, 2014, p. 6.

[97] U.S. Army Medical Command, 2014, p. 24.

- Potential Lesson: Clearly define program goals and design the program structure around those goals. Program goals should directly drive how the program should be set up and the principles that govern it.

- **Understanding specific unit needs and culture is critical.** This leads to trust, which is a critical factor: Providers must earn the trust of both the commanders and the service members by understanding their profession, spending substantial time with the unit, and being trained on the specific cultural factors as they relate to the unit and the service. Understanding unit mission needs means providers can better assess individuals' readiness to perform their jobs.

  - Potential Lesson: Train providers in unit-specific topics and culture, including the roles and responsibilities of individuals and the unit overall, so that trust can be built between providers and unit members and readiness can be assessed adequately.

- **Chain of command and organizational structure matters.** The Army's EBH team feels that the structure it uses, in which the providers are in the chain of command of the MTF but have a habitual relationship with the unit, is most effective because the provider can provide objective feedback without fear of retribution.

  - Potential Lesson: Structure the organizational chain of command specifically in line with program goals.

Navy (Embedded Mental Health)

History

The Navy has been using embedded mental health and physical health professionals since the mid-1990s, although the early efforts were not designed as part of an official embedded health program, and the Embedded Mental Health (EMH) program today retains characteristics that reflect its decentralized roots. Interviewees we spoke with noted that active duty mental health professionals were aboard the USS *Constellation* for a two-week period in 1996, effectively serving as an embedded team on that ship.[98] During a 1998–1999 deployment to the Persian Gulf, a U.S. Navy clinical psychologist and a psychiatric technician served on the USS *Carl Vinson* and reported to the USS *Carl Vinson* as permanent members of the ship's company. This was part of an "evolving health care doctrine" that was referred to at the time as Force Health Protection, and it was viewed as providing an "effective, beneficial, and cost-saving landmark improvement in providing quality medical care to the fleet."[99] During the same deployment, a Navy physical therapist and a physical therapy technician were also on board the USS *Carl Vinson*, and there were indications that their presence led to fewer visits to sick call for musculoskeletal problems and fewer evacuations compared with similar carrier deployments.[100]

---

[98] RAND interview with Navy EMH personnel, March 15, 2019.

[99] Wood, Koffman, and Arita, 2003.

[100] Ziemke, Koffman, and Wood, 2001.

Other pilot programs in this time frame have emerged in the Navy, including in the Navy Expeditionary Combat Command (NECC) and in certain submarine units, which will be described later in this section. Overall, the Navy's embedded health programs can be characterized as "bottom-up," or designed and implemented on a pilot basis in different units among several of the Navy's communities, which resulted in high levels of differentiation in the service's embedded programs. Because of the Navy's long experience with embedded health providers, in some quarters they are simply considered members of the unit's team rather than "extra" professionals who have been added to the unit.[101]

Navy Embedded Mental Health Structure

EMH in the Navy is viewed as a multidisciplinary effort in which mental health providers and behavioral health technicians (BHTs) work closely with operational unit and command leadership to meet the goal of increasing mission readiness.[102]

Management of EMH in the Navy is decentralized, in the sense that individual units have a lot of independence in implementing the program, and while there is currently limited overall guidance on the "theory of change" for the program, it can be considered to be an element of the Combat Operational Stress Control program (COSC).[103]

COSC is built on the idea of a military culture of "strong communal support generated from being part of a unit,"[104] and a component of COSC is the stress continuum model, which helps leaders view team member needs based on their levels of stress.[105] As Koffman et al. found in the deployment of the USS *Carl Vinson*, embedded health providers

> are in the unique position of being able to identify problems at early stages in the [stress continuum model]. By staying abreast of morale and remaining vigilant about the level of stress among unit personnel, carrier psychologists can intervene before problems become severe, either by reaching out to individuals or groups at particularly high risk for mental health problems, or by advising the command on policies to enhance a unit's overall psychological readiness. For many psychological disorders, most notably PTSD, early identification and treatment is essential to avoiding long-term difficulties.[106]

---

[101] RAND interview with Navy EMH personnel, March 15, 2019. Some carrier commanders were "almost offended" because calling their EMH personnel "embedded" made them sound less integral to the unit.

[102] RAND interview with Navy EMH personnel, March 15, 2019.

[103] Described in OPNAV Instruction 6520.1A, *Operational Stress Control Program* (Chief of Naval Operations, 2016).

[104] This according to Captain Paul S. Hammer, the director of the Defense Centers of Excellence for Psychological Health and Traumatic Brain Injury, as discussed in Naval Center for Combat and Operational Stress Control (2013).

[105] The stress continuum model describes four levels of stress indicated by the four "colors zones": ready (green), reacting (yellow), injured (orange), and ill (red). See Nash (2006) and Naval Center for Combat and Operational Stress Control (2013).

[106] Koffman et al., 2006, p. 126.

NECC implemented an EMH pilot program in 2010 in response to the need for embedded assets with the explosive ordnance disposal community. The success of the pilot led to its expansion in 2012 to the Naval Construction Group and to the rest of NECC forces in 2015.[107] In 2012, psychiatrists began routinely deploying with amphibious ready groups, and in 2015 a psychiatrist billet was created within fleet surgical teams.[108]

Finally, after starting with a pilot program in 2013 in response to the fact that 30 percent of all decreases to the submarine force were due to mental health diagnoses,[109] Submarine Force, U.S. Pacific Fleet, established the embedded Mental Health Program (eMHP),[110] the goal of which is to give sailors and personnel attached to Submarine Force, U.S. Pacific Fleet, command access to effective mental health care with the expectation of returning patients to "full duty."[111]

Even though management of EMH is decentralized in the Navy, efforts are underway to provide more guidance for the provision of these services. In early 2017, the Navy chartered the EMH clinical subcommunity with the goal of developing and disseminating clinical, operational, and business best practices and training requirements. Representation in the subcommunity includes Navy mental health specialty leaders, deckplate leaders,[112] type commanders, and marine expeditionary force surgeons. Major products of this effort include a 2017 laydown of EMH assets,[113] provider and leader surveys, and platform-specific guidebooks. The guidebooks equip incoming EMH providers with knowledge about the platform and best practices. Guidebooks have been completed for the submarine and surface warfare communities, a draft guidebook for the carrier community has recently been completed, and guidebooks for the Marine Corps and NECC are currently in development. Additionally, a working group under the EMH clinical subcommunity was recently established to identify the knowledge, skills, and abilities necessary to be successful in an EMH billet.

---

[107] See Kade, 2013.

[108] RAND interview with Navy EMH personnel, March 15, 2019; COMNECC/COMNECCPAC Instruction 1754.1C on the Family Readiness Program (Commander, Navy Expeditionary Combat Command, and Commander, Navy Expeditionary Combat Command Pacific, 2015) notes that a Family Readiness Council established to run the program will include the Force Embedded Mental Health Program Director.

[109] See Shenbergerhess (2019).

[110] The Submarine Force appears to use the abbreviation *eMHP* rather than *EMH*. See Miletich (2017).

[111] Miletich, 2017.

[112] Deckplate leaders include chief petty officers, work center supervisors, leading petty officers, and division officers (according to the Navy's *Command Resilience Team Guide* [U.S. Navy, Director, 21st Century Sailor Office (N17), 2018]).

[113] This laydown broke down the number of billets by platform (e.g., submarine forces, carriers, U.S. Marine Corps), provider type, ratio of service member to provider/unit and region, among other things. In October 2018, a revised comprehensive laydown of EMH in the Navy and Marine Corps was expanded to include all mental health resources available to line commanders.

Importantly, in 2017 the EMH clinical subcommunity created a logic model to visually represent the EMH program and its theory of change.[114] This model maps the relationships among various EMH inputs, activities, and outputs, resulting in short-, medium-, and long-term outcomes. In addition, the Navy Bureau of Medicine and Surgery, in coordination with line commanders, recently completed the development of an algorithm to determine ideal staffing that accounts for current resources, line commander requirements, and force generation differences between provider types.

Current Implementation and Team Composition

An EMH asset is generally an active duty mental health professional (officer or enlisted) who is directly attached to expeditionary commands and whose primary duties are to provide direct mental health support (e.g., direct clinical care, command liaison/consultation, outreach, education and training, psychological surveillance) to an expeditionary force or command. EMH teams include active duty psychiatrists, psychologists, LCSWs, psychiatric mental health nurse practitioners, and BHTs that are embedded and fully integrated into operational units.[115] According to the Navy's Surgeon General, embedded mental health providers in 2018 represented 25 percent of the Department of the Navy's mental health officer billets and roughly the same percentage for all enlisted BHT billets.[116]

The composition of embedded teams varies with the needs of the operational unit and requirements of the Navy Type Command. For example,[117]

- the submarine community has one psychologist and one BHT at each submarine concentration area.
- fleet surgical teams, which deploy with amphibious readiness groups, include one psychiatrist and one BHT.
- NECC has one LCSW at various NECC concentration areas.
- the Naval Air Forces has one psychologist and one BHT assigned to each aircraft carrier.

The surface Navy is adding different combinations of mental health professionals to provide comprehensive support to various fleet concentration areas based on the size of the concentration area, existing resources, and other variables. Deployment practices of the teams also vary with the billet. Specifically, the following EMH billets routinely deploy with the unit:

- fleet surgical team EMH

---

[114] RAND interview with Navy EMH personnel, March 15, 2019.

[115] RAND interview with Navy EMH personnel, March 15, 2019. Since 1983, the Navy has also used Special Psychiatric Rapid Intervention Teams (SPRINTs) (Koffman et al., 2006). SPRINT provides short-term mental health support to a requesting command shortly after a traumatic event with the goals of preventing long-term psychiatric dysfunction and promoting maximum psychological readiness. See the Navy Medical SPRINT site (Navy Medical Forces Atlantic, undated).

[116] Faison, 2018.

[117] RAND interview with Navy EMH personnel, March 15, 2019.

- aircraft carrier EMH
- some NECC EMH.

The following may deploy with their unit:

- Marine Corps EMH
- some NECC EMH.

And the following are in shore billets and are not expected to deploy:

- waterfront surface Navy EMH
- submarine EMH.

As mentioned above, management of EMH in the Navy is decentralized. As one interviewee told us, "We don't have a program—we have multiple programs operated by different line commands."[118] The same interviewee added, "one thing has become sacred: They are in control of their templates. . . . They don't want a centralized Navy system." This means that the command itself owns the billet, which creates inherent valuation of the program. It also provides the commanding officer control over the EMH asset, as opposed to sharing it with an MTF, which can allow for greater focus on the unit's needs.

Decentralized management also has drawbacks: For example, requirements are determined at the line level and requests for funding go through the appropriate channels within those units, so tracking the cost of the various programs is difficult. Further, assessing the various programs is difficult because there are no common metrics that are shared across units. However, the Chief of Naval Operations is creating a "data reservoir" as a central repository of information on certain behaviors. Finally, while decentralization allows a unit to tailor the program to its specific needs, it can inhibit sharing and adoption of best practices and lessons learned across commands as well.

Lessons the Air Force Can Learn from the Navy

- **Chain of command design matters.** In the Navy, line commanders own the embedded provider billets, not the MTFs.
  - Potential Lesson: Who the embedded providers report to (in the military chain of command versus belonging to an MTF) can have a major impact on how a service member accesses a provider, how familiar providers are with the unit, what diagnoses would be career enders for a particular unit's members, and how much trust commanders puts into what the providers tell them. Organizational design can also affect the degree to which service members are willing to be open with providers (for example, if a provider is in the chain of command, they might be compelled to share sensitive information with the commander, whereas a provider outside the chain of command would not have to).

---

[118] RAND interview with Navy program managers, March 22, 2019.

- **Be prepared to iterate and tailor programs to community needs.** The Navy's EMH efforts are not just one program, but rather a collection of programs that have been created based on demand, changing conditions, and lessons learned.
  - Potential Lesson: Consider whether centralized management of all programs and increased standardization should be prioritized or whether a more flexible, decentralized model is better given program goals.
- **Headquarters functions can help facilitate information-sharing about demand for specific training in manning, rather than generating strict and centralized guidelines or program management.**
  - Potential Lesson: A coordinating headquarters element can provide a useful purpose without exercising rigid standardization if it is not needed—for example by leading efforts to develop doctrine and training materials for the program.
- **The EMH program staff is currently working with different communities within the Navy to identify and record different programs' operations to institutionalize, though not standardize, efforts and lessons learned.**
  - Potential Lesson: Some degree of institutionalization is needed to track lessons learned and program effectiveness, and likely can occur without losing the flexibility that is needed to address different communities needs.
- **Lack of Navy program centralization means lack of centralized data.** The Navy is currently attempting to routinize and centralize some data collection to augment program effectiveness.
  - Potential Lesson: Programs do not need to be centralized and standardized, but data collection might need to be.

U.S. Marine Corps (Operational Stress Control and Readiness)

History

The Operational Stress Control and Readiness (OSCAR) concept was piloted in 1999 when the 2d Marine Division at Camp Lejeune, North Carolina, sought a new "type of partnership between warfighters and mental health professionals."[119] OSCAR's goal was to embed mental health personnel directly in operational units at the level of the regiment instead of attaching them to external MTFs or external combat stress teams. OSCAR psychiatrists, psychologists, and psychiatric technicians were organic to the units they supported, trained with their marines prior to deployment, and accompanied them during deployment.[120] As William Nash, formerly of the Headquarters, Marine Corps Office of Manpower and Reserve Affairs, described in 2006,

---

[119] Nash, 2006.

[120] Nash, 2006.

OSCAR builds a bridge across the cultural gap between warfighter and mental health professional the only way such a bridge can be built—by drawing the mental health professional as fully as possible into the culture and life of the military unit to be supported. As one commander of a Marine infantry battalion said to his newly assigned OSCAR psychiatrist, "I am never going to live in your world, so it's a good thing that you are here to learn about mine."[121]

In 2004, the Marine Corps, together with the Navy Bureau of Medicine, initiated a two-year pilot of OSCAR across all three active Marine Corps divisions.[122] A 2006 study of OSCAR conducted by the Center for Naval Analyses (CNA) found that it was reaching the desired target audiences and achieving desired outputs, so expansion of the program was recommended.[123] This led to a 2007 decision to request that OSCAR teams be available in the infantry divisions and regiments of all three marine expeditionary forces.[124] According to Koffman et al., "A formal request for OSCAR staffing was sent by the Marine Corps to the Navy in early 2008. Within a few months, the Navy approved funding to permanently staff OSCAR in the Marine divisions and regiments, both active and reserve, starting in 2010."[125]

From 2009 to 2016, OSCAR evolved to include three programs: OSCAR-P (P for "Provider"), which included mental health providers and psychiatric technicians in ground combat element regiments, became a program of record in 2009. OSCAR-M (M for "Mentor") training started in 2011 for a subset of noncommissioned officers (NCOs), senior NCOs, chaplains, and general medical officers in each battalion-sized unit, and in 2016 marine logistics groups (MLGs) acquired mental health assets for the provision of organic psychological care to their units.[126]

U.S. Marine Corps OSCAR Structure

OSCAR and COSC became strongly linked during Operations Iraqi Freedom and Enduring Freedom, and a 2007 COSC conference led to the development of Marine Corps and Navy COSC doctrine published in 2010 as *Combat and Operational Stress Control*.[127] According to this publication,

---

[121] Nash, 2006.

[122] Koffman et al., 2006, p. 127.

[123] The CNA study is quoted to this effect in Koffman et al. (2006), and the assessment was confirmed in our interviews with interviewees, but we could not obtain a copy of the CNA report.

[124] RAND interview with Navy EMH personnel, March 15, 2019.

[125] Koffman et al., 2006, p. 127.

[126] RAND interview with Navy EMH personnel, March 15, 2019. The OSCAR-M program appears to be the most studied, including a 2015 RAND study (Vaughan et al., 2015) and the 2006 CNA study quoted by Koffman et al., 2006. Interviewees told us that the programs are fragmented and incompletely implemented.

[127] U.S. Marine Corps, 2010.

Psychiatrists, psychologists, and psychiatric technicians who are part of the OSCAR program are organic to the military units they support in the same way battalion surgeons, corpsmen, and chaplains are organic to their Marine operational units. Ideally, OSCAR MHPs [mental health professionals] train with their Marines prior to deployment, accompany their Marines into forward operational areas during deployment, and continue to provide support to their Marines after they return from deployment. The OSCAR program bridges the cultural gap between warfighters and mental health professionals by drawing professionals as fully as possible into the culture and life of the military units they support and making them more members of the "family" than outsiders. The intent of this effort is to reduce the stigma of mental health care through familiarity and shared adversity.[128]

Follow-on guidance appeared in a marine administration message in 2011 that provided guidance on OSCAR requirements, team composition, and team roles, training, certification and reporting, and in a Marine Corps Order issued in February 2013.[129]

According to some we interviewed, there is little consistency in how OSCAR is implemented across the Marine Corps, and a commander can largely use the assets as they individually desire. One interviewee noted, "When commanders don't appreciate the mental health assets, they get used like MTF providers."[130] A criticism we heard was that there is no program manager for OSCAR, which can create issues in ensuring quality control in training and implementation across the service, and there is pressure from MTF commanders to have personnel in newly filled OSCAR billets work for the MTF instead of the unit commanders, as intended.[131]

Current Implementation and Team Composition

According to *Combat and Operational Stress Control*, OSCAR-M mentor teams are formed at the battalion level (units of approximately 1,000 marines) across the Marine Corps.[132] Each unit trains a team of approximately 50 OSCAR mentors, derived from both the battalion headquarters unit and subordinate units, and uses supporting extenders and mental health professionals from internal or local sources, as available. OSCAR "mentors" are trained marines within a particular unit, whereas OSCAR "extenders" are unit medical and religious ministry personnel.[133]

OSCAR-P mental health personnel include

psychiatrists, psychologists, mental health nurse practitioners, and licensed clinical social workers embedded in operational units to provide formal mental

---

[128] U.S. Marine Corps, 2010, Appendix N.

[129] U.S. Marine Corps, 2011, 2013.

[130] Interview, April 2, 2019.

[131] Vaughan et al., 2015.

[132] U.S. Marine Corps, 2010.

[133] U.S. Marine Corps, 2013, p. 2.1.

health services. The individuals assigned or invited to be part of the battalion team also depend on the type of unit and support available. Each infantry division generally includes three mental health professionals and four psychological technicians on their table of organization. Each infantry regiment typically includes two mental health professionals and two psychological technicians, all available on a shared basis to their respective battalions.[134]

The original OSCAR model fielded an interdisciplinary team of mental health professionals, experienced senior NCOs, and chaplains, but with the start of Operations Iraqi Freedom and Enduring Freedom, senior NCOs became too scarce a resource to include. According to interviewees, as of mid-2019, OSCAR structure includes the following:[135]

- Marine Corps Ground Combat Element: one psychologist, one psychiatrist, one social worker, and three BHTs that cover a regiment-sized unit
- Marine Corps Logistics Combat Element: two psychiatrists, two psychologists, and two BHTs within medical battalions, although the Marine Corps is planning to replicate the ground combat element model.

Generally, OSCAR-P personnel—the ones assigned to the regiment—will deploy if the regiment deploys. OSCAR-M mentors are NCOs already assigned to a unit, so they will deploy according to the unit's schedule. MLG OSCAR personnel are currently assigned to the medical battalion level. The medical battalion is a unit within a logistics group, so MLG OSCAR personnel will deploy only if the medical battalion deploys with the unit.[136]

Lessons the Air Force Can Learn from the Marine Corps

The Marine Corps experiences with embedded mental health providers offer several lessons for the Air Force.

- **Create a mechanism to coordinate across programs.** Three disparate OSCAR programs exist, and the efforts of the programs have historically been largely separate.

  - Potential Lesson: if multiple types of programs exist, a mechanism should be created to ensure communication is intact, so gaps and unnecessary redundancies are addressed.

- **Lack of institutionalization can lead to incomplete implementation.** Very little program institutionalization or standardization exists, including no doctrinal codification, despite OSCAR being a program of record since 2009. Because of this lack of

---

[134] U.S. Marine Corps, 2010, Appendix N.

[135] Our research was completed in 2019. For a 2020 update on the structure of the Ground Combat Element and Logistics Combat Element, see Katherine E. Pierce, David Broderick, Scott Johnston, Kathryn J. Holloway, "Embedded Mental Health in the United States Marine Corps," *Military Medicine*, Vol. 185, Nos. 9–10, September– October 2020.

[136] Interview with U.S. Marine Corps personnel, April 2, 2019.

institutionalization, program implementation is not complete, and program effectiveness is difficult to measure.

- – Potential Lesson: Without institutionalization and DOTMLPF-P (doctrine, organization, training, materiel, leadership and education, personnel, facilities, and policy) implementation, programs will be incompletely implemented and difficult to assess.

- **Holistic mental health assessments are critical.** Marines are assessed both by mental health providers and trained NCOs. This can allow disparate perceptions to be resolved and for understanding of specific unit requirements to have weight in decisions about mental health readiness. This model also has drawbacks, as factors such as stigma or unit readiness priorities can be injected into the process through the NCO's assessment.

- – Potential Lesson: Holistic, multisource assessments can provide value, especially when compiled from multiple perspectives, including one or more that understands the service members' unique roles.
- – Potential Lesson: Cultural training and familiarity for the providers are essential to gaining trust and understanding of service members' needs.

- **Centralized program management is needed to create accountability and consistency across the program.** OSCAR overall is highly varied in management and implementation and tailored to what an individual commander wants. This means that the commander's education about OSCAR is largely up to the provider, and it is very difficult to implement the program with any consistency.

- – Potential Lesson: Centralized program management of some kind is needed to create responsibility, ensure that the overall mission is matched with the organization that provides the manpower, and create communication and continuity between programs. Further, some sort of oversight body can help the service advocate for needed changes and increased funding and can help foster data collection on program effectiveness and share lessons learned among different units.

- **Expand access to embedded care as needed.** OSCAR was originally designed to focus on ground combat units, but over time the Marine Corps noted high demand for embedded care in logistics and aviation career fields and expanded the access accordingly to those communities.

- – Potential Lesson: Supporting the perceived high-risk unit might not be enough, and program managers should be open to expanding embedded care access to other populations and making other program changes based on lessons learned in implementation.

U.S. Special Operations Command (Preservation of the Force and Family)

History

The ideas underlying the Preservation of the Force and Family (POTFF) initiative came from Admiral Eric T. Olson, commander of USSOCOM in 2011. According to his successor, Admiral William H. McRaven,

> My predecessor . . . initiated a Pressure on the Force and Families (POTFF) study to examine the effects of a decade of continuous combat operations on the SOF community. The study identified core problems, their underlying factors, and captured best practices of Service and SOF support programs. The research included more than 400 non-attribution focus groups, consisting of more than 7,000 service members and more than 1,000 spouses from 55 different SOF units located at home and overseas. The results of the study illustrated two primary sources of ongoing stress. First is the lack of predictability resulting from a demanding operational tempo, exacerbated by significant time spent away from home for training. Second is an increased difficulty for our force when reconnecting and reintegrating into family activities.[137]

Based on the findings of that study, McRaven directed his staff to transition the Pressure on the Force and Families Task Force to the Preservation of the Force and Families Task Force. His intent was not just a name change; he wanted to develop

> innovative solutions across the SOCOM enterprise to improve the well-being of our force and families. While we understand that this begins with increasing predictability, the holistic approach will also ensure we provide responsive counseling, medical, psychological, and rehabilitative care to our SOF warriors and their families.[138]

Therefore, the POTFF program is on one hand a set of formal programs but, on the other, an overarching concept that is intended to demonstrate commitment to addressing these issues. This two-sided definition is fundamental to understanding the nature of the POTFF embedded health efforts.

U.S. Special Operations Command POTFF Structure

Formal policy guidance for POTFF is limited, in part because USSOCOM endeavors to allow the program to be as tailored to operational unit needs as possible, and because its service component commands and Joint Special Operations Command forces all come from different services and backgrounds and are geared toward varied mission sets. According to the USSOCOM POTFF website, the mission of POTFF is

> to build and implement a holistic approach to address the pressure on our force. The POTFF-TF [Task Force] will identify and implement innovative, valuable

---

[137] McRaven, 2012.

[138] McRaven, 2012.

solutions across the USSOCOM Enterprise aimed at improving the short and long-term well-being of our SOF warriors and their families.[139]

POTFF addresses four "domains":[140]

- *psychological performance*, designed to improve the cognitive and behavioral performance of the force
- *human performance*, to meet the unique physical needs of SOF operators with holistic, embedded treatment and training
- *social and family performance*, which incorporates family resilience programs designed to enhance service-provided programs
- *spiritual performance*, which is designed to enhance core spiritual beliefs, values, awareness, relationships, and experiences.

However, lack of formal policy guidance has not prevented USSOCOM leadership from strongly supporting the program and requiring elements of the program at the O-6 level, and sometimes below.

Current Implementation and Team Composition

POTFF has a centralized requirements and procurement policy but a decentralized approach to execution, meaning that the program is highly tailored to individual units, given high variance in unit composition, mission areas, and deployment type.[141] The vast majority of POTFF providers are contractors; the initial POTFF contract (awarded to Booz Allen Hamilton, Inc., in 2013) paid for more than 300 contractors in the categories of sports psychologists, physical therapists, strength and conditioning specialists, LCSWs, and nurse case managers.[142] When the contract was re-competed in 2018, the Performance Work Statement called for personnel in 16 categories and planned to fund 505 positions at 37 locations from fiscal year (FY) 2019 to FY 2021.[143]

How the actual distribution of personnel is determined is unclear; however, POTFF "conducts an annual needs assessment survey to identify and address issues and stressors

---

[139] See USSOCOM (2019).

[140] Domains and descriptions are also from USSOCOM (2019).

[141] RAND interview with POTFF personnel.

[142] Koufas, 2016.

[143] USSOCOM, *Performance Work Statement (PWS), Preservation of the Force and Family (POTFF) Programs Support Contract*, March 12, 2018. The personnel types are (1) Biostatistician/Operations Research and System Analyst Support Specializing in Human Performance Consulting, (2) Certified Athletic Trainer, (3) Clinical Psychologist, (4) Cognitive Performance Specialist, (5) Community Program and Peer Network Coordinator (CPPNC), (6) Community Program Peer Network Coordinator Component Headquarters Advisor (CPPNC-CHA), (7) Data Scientist I, (8) Family Support Coordinator, (9) Human Performance Advisor, (10) Licensed Clinical Social Worker, (11) Nurse Case Manager, (12) Operational Psychologist, (13) Performance Dietician, (14) Physical Therapist, (15) Psychological/Mental Health Technician, and (16) Strength and Conditioning Specialist.

affecting the force and their families."[144] According to interviews, every USSOCOM unit has POTFF capabilities, and recently the USSOCOM commander mandated that human performance and psychological performance capabilities be embedded at each unit. There is some guidance on how the provider packages should be tailored to units depending on who composes them: Operators (Tier 1) have the most intensive resources available, enablers (Tier 2) follow, and other support personnel, such as headquarters personnel (Tier 3), are third.[145] USSOCOM found that simply providing POTFF resources to operators, which was the original design, left critical members of the team that support SOF operators behind. As one interviewee noted to us, "Special operators of course have specific demands, physically and psychologically, but we have found that your key enablers and your people need to be physically and psychologically able or the unit will fail. We can't have one group of people having this and one not."[146]

According to interviews, although the POTFF personnel work for the commander and, conceptually, everyone is embedded as a single team, they depend on the local MTF for quality assurance. Typically, POTFF providers do not deploy, although there have been occasions where they have done so on a short-term basis. There are also organic behavioral health providers for many units—uniformed personnel that are considered part of POTFF because their services can be leveraged for POTFF purposes. They deploy, but as military personnel they are not funded through the POTFF contract.

Lessons the Air Force Can Learn from the POTFF Program

- **Implementing an embedded health program without a full plan and articulated goals can create problems later, although there is benefit to building flexibility into the model so it can be iterated in the future.** USSOCOM's original data collection methods were not centralized, which has been challenging both internally and in justifying the program externally.

  - Potential Lesson: Articulate goals at the onset of the program and design the program to support those goals.
  - Potential Lesson: Design and implement a standardized data collection process up front so that analysis of program effectiveness and needed changes can be facilitated.
  - Potential Lesson: Be prepared to tailor the program and iterate as needed, whether by opening the program to different types of units, including additional or different providers, or increasing or decreasing standardization.

- **POTFF received strong, high-level attention and buy-in early as the USSOCOM commander advocated for it as his top priority.** This has been necessary to maintain

---

[144] See USSOCOM (2019).

[145] In interviews, we were told that this is described in a POTFF policy memo, but we have not seen a copy of the memo.

[146] RAND interview with POTFF personnel.

momentum, receive funding, and ensure buy-in from all different types of commands in the organization.

- – Potential Lesson: Ensure that attention is driven from the highest command leadership levels down through the command so that the program receives proper advocacy, funding, and focus.

- **Work across different program focus areas.** The formal POTFF program has four domains: physical, psychological, social, spiritual. Recent guidance has mandated that all units have a program that addresses the first two. Despite the different providers needed for each of those domains, all teams work together as one.

  - – Potential Lesson: Different focus areas for embedded providers can still mean collaboration and a team-oriented approach to the collective goal of providing needed care along a range of health and readiness issues.

- **POTFF has a centralized procurement policy and requirements component, but a decentralized implementation side given the specialized needs of all the different units under USSOCOM.**

  - – Potential Lesson: An embedded program can effectively have both centralized management and tailorable and decentralized implementation.
  - – Potential Lesson: Programs can be tailored to an individual unit's needs so long as there is an overarching goal and program management that ties the programs together.

- **All personnel, from the warfighter to headquarters support personnel, receive some level of POTFF support.** Originally focused just on the warfighter, USSOCOM realized that enablers and support personnel also needed to be in peak health for the mission to be accomplished, so adjusted the model. Not everyone receives the same packages and treatment, but everyone has access to some level of the program.

  - – Potential Lesson: Supporting only the highest-risk units and personnel might be insufficient to achieve mission goals and desired readiness levels.
  - – Potential Lesson: The type and the density of providers can be modified depending on the needs of the personnel that compose a particular unit, but a standard baseline should exist for certain types of providers, depending on the needs of the service.

- **Virtually all contracted providers have a military and SOF background.** This helps to ensure familiarity with unit needs, and breeds trust with unit personnel.

  - – Potential Lesson: Train providers in understanding unit culture and roles.

- **Key point: The physically embedded teams, and the frequency of their interactions with the unit, are critical to the success of POTFF.** Providers who are easy to access and who are perceived as part of the unit are key to trust and utilization.

  - – Potential Lesson: Embed the providers to the greatest extent possible, fostering frequent interaction and communication, to ensure access.

Conclusion

Though not exhaustive, our analysis of the embedded health programs in the Army, Navy, Marine Corps, and USSOCOM shows that each service administers its program in ways substantially different than the others. For example, the degree of standardization among the programs ranges from very little, as is the case with USSOCOM's POTFF program, to highly standardized, as in the Army's EBH program. Further, organizational structure, chain of command, and the personnel included in provider teams also varies widely among the other services and USSOCOM. Each program demonstrates its own strengths and trade-offs and can offer critical lessons for the Air Force's efforts.

Despite variations in program design and implementation, through interviews with program stakeholders, we identified some key commonalities that characterize the other services' and USSOCOM's programs:

- First and foremost, program design must follow directly from program goals, rather than the inverse. The type of specific program goal of the embedded program—for example, to increase readiness, to provide better medical care for the service member, to strengthen relationships between providers and units—will directly affect how the program should be structured, whether providers should fall within the unit chain of command, and how data on program effectiveness should be collected.
- Second, all embedded providers need to be able to build trust and buy-in with both unit commanders and service members. Interviewees we spoke with emphasized two key elements in forging those relationships: (1) effective training in and/or underlying understanding of specific unit needs and unit and service culture and (2) actual embedding within the units to increase repeat interactions, increase accessibility, and normalize treatment so that stigma is lessened. Further, each interviewee stressed that the providers need to understand the unit's responsibilities and unique characteristics in order to be able to correctly determine whether a service member is fit for duty.
- Third, even if programs are not centralized or standardized across all units, data collection should be centralized so that the service can better disseminate lessons learned, have adequate information to effectively advocate for additional resources, and better target efforts to address program goals whether in specific units or across the service's program.

Chapter 4. RAND Framework for Squadron Risks, Development of Personnel Packages, and Assessments of Costs

The goal of TFTN is to increase Air Force readiness. By embedding and improving access to "helping" agencies, such as mental health teams, religious support teams, and physical health teams, the Air Force hopes to reduce systemic squadron risk, leverage installations' existing community support infrastructure, increase help-seeking behavior by airmen, better connect airmen to services, and make better use of evidence-based interpersonal and self-directed violence prevention tools.[147]

In this chapter, we describe the framework that we developed independently to identify risk levels of squadrons in order to prioritize the provision of TFTN teams. We then discuss the composition of provider teams that we developed independently to assist squadrons at risk. Then we present the approach that we used to determine the potential personnel costs of TFTN teams for FYs 2020 through 2025, based on our independent risk framework and the personnel packages that we developed.

It is important to note that our framework served as the basis for the Air Force's TFTN team's assessment of risk across Air Force squadrons. We suggested additional data sources that the Air Force could access to strengthen the RAND framework. Ultimately, the Air Force was able to access additional sensitive data sources (e.g., suicide data, sexual assault data) to build on the RAND framework and create a more robust data set. Similarly, our initial personnel packages served as a foundation for the Air Force's TFTN team's final personnel packages. The TFTN team adjusted our personnel packages in response to the program's evolving goals and priorities. Therefore, although the Air Force's final analyses differ from our initial findings, this chapter serves to document the approach and findings of our initial analysis.

RAND Framework and Assessment of Squadron Risk Factors

Data and Metrics Used for Initial RAND Risk Framework and Assessments

The first step that we took in determining a squadron's risk and its need for assistance in any of the CAF domains was to establish some measures of the current status of each domain. To do so, we made use of data and approaches developed by the AFRL/711th HPW, detailed data from the Air Force's MilPDS, and analyses from earlier RAND research. These data sources enabled us to develop risk metrics for the physical, mental, and social domains. Given the lack of available data, we were unable to develop any metrics for the spiritual domain.

---

[147] Robinson, 2019b.

711th Human Performance Wing

As part of the Air Force's effort to "revitalize" squadrons, in 2018 the Air Force Medical Service developed the concept of operational support teams (OSTs), which are provider teams that would rotate through squadrons at a base and provide programs to improve individual health and squadron performance.[148]

To prioritize the provision of OST services, the AFRL developed a risk measure that uses "profile" data related to conditions that restrict the mobility or duty of individual airmen.[149] This profile information is maintained in the Aeromedical Services Information Management System (ASIMS) and includes codes related to an individual's mental health characteristics and musculoskeletal injuries. AFRL assumed that a unit with higher numbers of individuals "on profile" for mental health or musculoskeletal injury would be at higher risk of being less ready to deploy. AFRL developed unit profile risk scores for mental health and musculoskeletal injury based on a unit's deviation from the Air Force average, while accounting for unit size, with scores ranging from risk group 1 (RG1, highest risk) to risk group 5 (RG5, lowest risk).[150] The 711th HPW used a similar approach to develop a suicide risk measure for units. In neither case was RAND granted access to the underlying data that were used to determine the scores or rankings.[151]

We used the musculoskeletal injury risk score as an input for an assessment of risk in the CAF physical domain, and the mental health and suicide risk scores as inputs for the status of the mental domain.

Military Personnel Data System

The MilPDS includes extensive information in a variety of categories about military and civilian personnel assigned to Air Force units. We examined these variables for their potential association with risk in the physical domain (individuals who cannot be deployed because of a physical condition, for example) and the social domain (such as individuals who are exhibiting poor behavior) and selected those shown in Table 4.1. In the physical domain, for example, if MilPDS shows that an individual must be assigned to a base with a hospital, it is likely an indicator that the airman is not deployable. Also, deferment from deployment because of

---

[148] Holstein, 2018. As an example of support team composition, an OST that started at Joint Base Elmendorf-Richardson in June 2018 consisted of a physical therapist, a psychologist, two nutritionists, an exercise physiologist, and a human performance integrator technician.

[149] "Profiles are descriptions of transient or permanent limitations to functioning which are used for establishing suitability for career fields or Air Force Specialty Codes (AFSCs). A profile can be established on a DD Form 2808, Report of Medical Examination, an AF Form 422, or other forms as directed" (AFI 10-203, 2014, paragraph 1.2.2).

[150] See Appendix A for a description of the methodology.

[151] The scores were provided to RAND by the sponsor in an Excel spreadsheet named "All Major Installation Risk Group Distribution Data." The spreadsheet has musculoskeletal injury, mental health, and suicide risk rankings for individual units.

participation in the Exceptional Family Member Program (EFMP)[152] means that a dependent of an individual has special medical or educational needs; one reason we include it as an indicator of risk in the physical domain is that, in addition to being an indicator of nondeployability, it could be associated with a family member's need for the physical or medical assistance meant to be provided by TFTN.[153]

All the variables in the social domain category are meant to indicate the presence of negative social behaviors in a squadron. A large number of individuals in drug rehabilitation programs or with convictions of drug use, for example, could not only affect deployability, but also indicate problems with discipline or morale.

Table 4.1. MilPDS Indicators of Risk in the Physical and Social Domains

Indicators of Risk in the Physical Domain	Indicators of Risk in the Social Domain
Assignment limited to a base with a hospital	Unfavorable information file[b]
EFMP deferment[a]	Article 15
Humanitarian/permissive deferment	Court-martial
Medical or physical evaluation board	DEROS (date of earliest return from overseas)[c] denied for cause
Medically disqualified for deployment	Demotion or withheld promotion
Temporary medical deferment	Drugs (conviction or in rehabilitation)

[a] Having a dependent in the EFMP or needing a humanitarian deferment can cause stress for an individual. As noted in Chapter 2, stress can affect physical well-being. These factors are exploratory, and we recognize that they could be included in other domains.
[b] An unfavorable information file documents administrative, judicial, or non-judicial censures concerning the member's performance, responsibility, and behavior (see AFI 36-2907, 2014).
[c] Denial of DEROS can mean that an individual's overseas tour is being involuntarily extended because of an investigation for wrongdoing, court-martial, or completing an Article 15 action (see AFI 36-2110, 2018).

We developed a "nondeployable for physical reasons" variable that shows the percentage of military personnel in a squadron who were not deployable because of any of the six physical risk factors in the past five years. A "social detractor" variable was similarly developed, showing the percentage of military personnel in a squadron who had any of the social risk factors in the past five years.[154]

---

[152] The EFMP/Special Needs program is described at the USAF Services website (USAF Services, undated).

[153] EFMP also applies to families who need assistance with behavioral health and special education, so one might argue that it could be included as part of the mental health metric.

[154] Assignments tend to last three years. The five-year period was chosen to take into account the relative rarity of these factors and to account for the possibility that a factor in a previous assignment could affect an individual in their current assignment.

In early 2014, DoD asked the RAND National Defense Research Institute to conduct an independent assessment of sexual assault, sexual harassment, and gender discrimination in the military. This request led to the RAND Military Workplace Study, which from August to September 2014 conducted one of the largest surveys of its kind related to problems in the workplace: Almost 560,000 active- and reserve-component service members were invited to participate, and more than 170,000 completed the survey."[155]

One volume of the resulting report, *Sexual Assault and Sexual Harassment in the U.S. Military, Annex to Volume 5*, includes tables that estimate the average sexual assault or sexual harassment risk that service members experience at installations or major commands expressed as a percentage.[156] We used these risk percentages as an input to a squadron's risk in the social domain and assumed that all squadrons at an installation shared the same sexual assault risk.

Table 4.2 summarizes the data sources used and variables developed for our determination of squadron risk levels.

Table 4.2. Data Sources and Applicable CAF Domains

Data Source	Data Used and Applicable Domain
Aeromedical Services Information Management System (ASIMS)	Physical domain: musculoskeletal injury profile Mental domain: mental health profile
711th Human Performance Wing	Mental domain: suicide risk factor data
Sexual Assault and Sexual Harassment in the U.S. Military, Annex to Volume 5, Tables A.5 and A.6	Social domain: sexual assault prevalence
Military Personnel Data System (MilPDS)	Physical domain: nondeployability variable based on several other MilPDS variables Social domain: social "detractor" variable based on several other MilPDS variables

Establishing Squadron Risk Levels

For each of the variables described above, we ranked squadrons from most at-risk to least at-risk based on the percentage of people in the squadron who had a characteristic (in the case of MilPDS data), risk score (in the case of mental health, musculoskeletal injury, and suicide data), or the percentage level of risk (in the case of sexual assault). For each variable, we determined the percentile of the squadron relative to other squadrons.

Table 4.3 shows how the variables were combined to determine squadron risk levels in the physical, mental, and social domains.

---

[155] Morral, Gore, and Schell, 2016.

[156] Morral, Gore, and Schell, 2016. Table A.5 in the appendix shows sexual assault risk for women; Table A.6 shows sexual assault risk for men.

Table 4.3. Variables Used to Determine Initial Risk Levels in Each Domain

Domain	Risk Determination
Physical	Average of the squadron percentile for the MilPDS "non-deployable for physical reasons" variable and the unit percentile for musculoskeletal injury risk factor
Mental	Average of the squadron percentile for mental health risk factor and the unit percentile for suicide risk factor
Social	Average of the squadron percentile for the MilPDS social detractor variable, installation-level risk for female sexual assault, and installation-level risk for male sexual assault

The Air Force has more than 2,000 active duty squadrons. Although MilPDS includes data for all of them, data sources for some of the variables in Table 4.3 were more limited: There were 1,375 Air Force squadrons for which there was data on mental health risk, musculoskeletal injury risk, and sexual assault risk. Of these squadrons, 99 were missing data on suicide risk, and in these cases suicide risk was considered to be blank and was not included in any calculations.

After ranking squadrons in each domain, we categorized them as being at high, medium, and low risk in each domain as follows:

- High risk: top 5 percent of squadrons by risk
- Medium risk: the next 10 percent of squadrons
- Low risk: the remaining 85 percent of squadrons.

We decided on these cut points because of the low frequency of positive responses in the data: Most squadrons have few or zero people with a positive response, so any positive response automatically makes a squadron above average. With such skewed data, assigning the highest 5 percent as "High" and the next 10 percent as "Medium" is a prudent approach.

Analysis of Personnel Package Composition

We were not able to find any data on the relative effectiveness of one type of embedded provider versus another; therefore, we looked to the types of providers that are currently included in other examples of embedded provider programs. We strongly recommend that as the Air Force expands the TFTN program, it carefully track the effectiveness of the different types of providers included in the packages. In particular, if there is variation across the composition of the personnel packages, it is especially important to capture the difference in outcomes across those personnel packages.

The initial POTFF contract provided funding for up to 300 contractors in the categories of sports psychologists, physical therapists, and strength and conditioning specialists for the human performance category and LCSWs and nurse case managers in the social and family performance category.[157] However, although USSOCOM has had experience with POTFF since 2013, we

---

[157] See Koufas (2016), Holstein (2018); U.S. Air Force, 2017.

could find no information about how it determines the number of personnel needed at a given location, nor how it determines the most effective mix or ratio of embedded providers.

The Air Force provides at least two examples of the composition of teams needed to provide TFTN-related care. First, one of the initial Air Force OSTs established at Joint Base Elmendorf-Richardson in June 2018 consisted of six personnel: a physical therapist, a psychologist, two nutritionists, an exercise physiologist, and a human performance integrator technician.[158] Second, the request for proposal for the TFTN test program included physical therapists, exercise physiologists, human performance technicians, LCSWs, clinical psychologists, and mental health technicians.[159]

Table 4.4 compares the personnel types required by the three programs.

Table 4.4. Comparison of POTFF, OST, and TFTN Test Program Personnel Packages

Personnel Category	POTFF	Operational Support Teams	TFTN Program
LCSW	X		X
Nurse case manager	X		
Clinical psychologist		X	X
Mental health technician			X
Sports psychologist	X		
Physical therapist	X	X	X
Strength and conditioning coach	X		X
Exercise physiologist		X	X
Nutritionist		X	X
Human performance integrator technician		X	

SOURCES: Koufas, 2016; Holstein, 2018; U.S. Air Force, 2017.

Using these examples of the types of personnel required for similar embedded provider programs in the services, we determined that the personnel required for low-, medium-, and high-risk squadrons in the three domains are those displayed in Table 4.5. Note that there is a personnel type in Table 4.5 that is not in Table 4.4: community support coordinator. We added this personnel type to provide a liaison to other social support resources.

---

[158] See Holstein (2018).

[159] Draft solicitation number FA701417R1016, issue date October 5, 2017.

43

Table 4.5. Personnel Packages for Low-, Medium-, and High-Risk Squadrons

Personnel Category	Mental			Social			Physical		
	Low	Medium	High	Low	Medium	High	Low	Medium	High
LCSW	X	X	X		X	X			
Clinical psychologist			X			X			
Mental health technician	X	X	X						
Community support coordinator				X	X	X			
Physical therapist								X	X
Strength and conditioning coach									X
Performance nutritionist									X
Exercise physiologist									X

Although the composition of personnel packages was defined for the different risk levels by CAF domain, the categorization of the risk levels of each squadron allowed us to estimate the costs of providing these packages to squadrons that need them.

Estimate of Initial TFTN Personnel Packages

General Ground Rules and Assumptions

There were 1,375 squadrons for which RAND had access to data that could be used to identify a requirement for some level of TFTN support. Based on the squadron risk levels assigned to each squadron by domain (mental, social, and physical) and the personnel packages assigned to each domain, a total of 8,977 personnel would be required at full implementation. The baseline assumption was to include only military personnel and government civilians to fill the various positions identified in the personnel packages. Additional scenarios called for including contractor personnel, due primarily to the challenges of hiring a large number of people in a short amount of time, especially in areas requiring special skills.

Cost of RAND's Initial Independent Assessment of Providing TFTN Personnel Packages

General Ground Rules and Assumptions

The estimates below include only the costs of additional personnel. There will likely be other costs to consider, including facilities, equipment, and funds for unit activities. The assumptions and data were not available at this time to estimate or include these costs, as the focus of this report is on the personnel impacts.

Unless otherwise noted, all estimates were inflated to then year (TY) dollars using the Office of the Under Secretary of Defense (Comptroller)'s FY 2019 "Green Book."[160] For estimating purposes, we made assumptions with respect to the pay grade for each position. Rather than make assumptions regarding pay grade and time in service at the individual level, we used gross averages. For civilian personnel, we assumed a GS-14, step 5 pay grade. For officers, we assumed an O-3 with six years of service. For enlisted service members, we assumed an E-5 with eight years of service.

Military Personnel Cost Assumptions

For base pay, we used the 2019 military pay rate table for the base year estimate, with costs inflated in out years using the FY 2019 "Green Book." We used the 2019 Basic Allowance for Housing (BAH) and Overseas Housing Allowance rates to estimate housing costs. Using the list of squadrons, we adjusted these costs using the locality adjustment for each installation. Another factor affecting BAH rates is whether the service member has dependents. Without specific data, we made the assumption that 60 percent of officers have dependents and 40 percent of enlisted personnel have dependents at the respective pay grades. Finally, the Basic Allowance for Subsistence (BAS) is also based on the 2019 rates.

To capture the full cost of integrating new military members, we used the Office of the Secretary of Defense (OSD) Cost Assessment and Program Evaluation (CAPE) Full Cost of Manpower (FCoM) model.[161] This model allows us to estimate additional costs, which will be the responsibility of the specific component, the larger DoD, and the federal government. Table 4.6 summarizes the additional costs included in the military personnel cost estimates.

Table 4.6. Full Cost of Manpower Military Cost Categories

Component Costs	DoD Costs	Federal Government Costs
<ul><li>Retired pay accrual</li><li>Training</li><li>Permanent change of station/relocation</li><li>Miscellaneous expenses</li><li>Medicare-eligible retiree health care</li><li>Education assistance</li><li>Recruitment/advertising</li></ul>	<ul><li>Discount groceries</li><li>Child development (day care facilities)</li><li>DoD Education Activity and Family Assistance</li><li>Health care (active duty service member and active duty family member)</li></ul>	<ul><li>Child education (Impact Aid)</li><li>Treasury contribution for concurrent receipts</li><li>Treasury contribution for Medicare-Eligible Retiree Health Care Fund (MERHCF)</li><li>Veterans benefits (cash and in-kind)</li></ul>

---

[160] To account for inflation, we used the inflation indices in the Office of the Under Secretary of Defense (Comptroller) *National Defense Budget Estimates for FY 2019*, also known colloquially as the "Green Book" (Office of the Under Secretary of Defense [Comptroller], 2018).

[161] Detailed documentation on how the DoD CAPE FCoM model estimates the manpower costs for all military personnel and government civilians is available at the FCoM website (Office of the Secretary of Defense, Cost Assessment and Program Evaluation, 2020, Not available to the general public).

Government Civilian Personnel Cost Assumptions

For base pay, we used the 2019 General Schedule (GS) pay rate table for the base year estimate, with costs inflated in out years using the FY 2019 "Green Book." Additionally, unlike military base pay, GS base pay is adjusted based on location. Using the list of squadrons, we adjusted these costs using the locality adjustment for each installation.

Like the military compensation costs, we used the OSD CAPE FCoM model to include other compensation, including both component-related costs and federal government costs. Table 4.7 summarizes the additional costs included in the government civilian cost estimates.

Table 4.7. Full Cost of Manpower Government Civilian Cost Categories

Component Costs	Federal Government Costs
• Overtime/holiday/other pays • Incentive/performance awards • Retention allowance • Social Security and Medicare (employer's contribution) • Recruitment/relocation bonuses • Health care (employer's share under the Federal Employees Health Benefits Program) • Personal travel/permanent change of station • Federal Employee Group Life Insurance • Transportation subsidies • Worker's compensation payments • Retirement accrual (employer's contribution) • Federal Retirement Thrift Investment Board payments (Thrift Savings Plan matching) • Unemployment insurance payments (Federal Unemployment Tax Act) • Severance pay/separation incentive • Severance health benefit • Training	• Postretirement life insurance • Postretirement health benefit

FYs 2020–2025 Cost Summary

Table 4.8 summarizes the costs from FYs 2020 to 2025. The phasing assumptions of the costs come from an initial Program Objective Memorandum (POM) estimate completed by the Air Force for TFTN. Costs are shown by risk domain (social, physical, and mental) and military and civilian personnel.

46

Table 4.8. Cost Estimate Summary

Personnel Type	Risk Domain	FY 2020	FY 2021	FY 2022	FY 2023	FY 2024	FY 2025
Military	Social	$0	$105	$197	$226	$246	$251
	Physical	$0	$288	$537	$617	$671	$686
	Mental	$0	$231	$431	$495	$539	$550
Civilian	Social	$0	$6	$10	$12	$13	$13
	Physical	$0	$0	$0	$0	$0	$0
	Mental	$0	$5	$10	$12	$13	$13
Total		**$0**	**$635**	**$1,185**	**$1,361**	**$1,482**	**$1,513**

NOTES: All costs are in millions of TY dollars. Some numbers may not sum correctly because of rounding.

It is important to note that our risk levels and our personnel packages were quickly overcome by events: As the Air Force refined its goals for TFTN, the composition of the personnel packages changed, and as it acquired more data, the risk levels of squadrons also changed. We outline those changes in the next chapter.

Conclusion

In this chapter, we presented the framework that we developed for the Air Force's TFTN team to assist them in identifying the level of mental, physical, and social risk in squadrons, as well as the initial personnel packages that we developed for high-, medium-, and low-risk squadrons across the CAF domains. Our initial cost estimates and personnel packages presented in this chapter rapidly became overcome by events as the Air Force TFTN team refined its goals for the TFTN program. However, our squadron risk framework and initial squadron risk assessment and personnel packages served as a foundation for the Air Force's further assessments of risk and further development of the TFTN personnel packages. The TFTN team was able to access additional data sources suggested by RAND related to sensitive topics, such as sexual assault, suicide, and problematic behaviors, which allowed the Air Force to build an even more robust data set on risk metrics. We recommend that the Air Force continue to build on the framework that we developed and continue to acquire additional data to inform its evolving risk metrics.

Chapter 5. Alternative Courses of Action for Expanding TFTN

In the course of developing personnel packages and assessing squadron risks independently, the RAND team worked in collaboration with the Air Force to develop alternative options and develop associated cost estimates in an effort to examine the trade-offs between implementing robust embedded teams in a timely fashion with the reality of expected budgetary constraints. In this chapter, we discuss the Air Force's revised risk framework and revised personnel packages that were based on our independent analyses presented in the previous chapter, as well as the various alternative options for expanding TFTN, the assumptions associated with each option, and the resulting cost estimates.

The Air Force's Risk Framework and Personnel Packages

As the Air Force TFTN team refined its goals for the TFTN program and was able to gain access to additional data, the RAND squadron risk framework, and initial squadron risk assessment and personnel packages served as a foundation for the Air Force's further assessments of risk and further development of the TFTN personnel packages. Specifically, the TFTN team was able to access additional data sources suggested by RAND related to sensitive topics such as sexual assault, suicide, and problematic behaviors, which allowed the Air Force to build an even more robust data set on risk metrics. The cost analyses in the subsequent sections of this chapter are based on this revised risk framework and revised personnel packages.

Air Force Risk Framework

As a result of gaining access to additional data, the Air Force was ultimately able to access mental health and physical risk for 1,870 squadrons in the Air Force (495 more squadrons than the initial RAND analysis). In refining its risk assessment, the Air Force decided to focus only on assessing mental and physical risk. The Air Force also added a fourth risk level (high+) to designate those squadrons that it identified as most at-risk and, therefore, priorities for receiving TFTN resources. As a result, the personnel packages also changed.

Air Force Mental and Physical Health Personnel Packages by Squadron Risk Level

The Air Force personnel packages for each mental health (MH) and physical health (PH) risk level are summarized in Tables 5.1 and 5.2. There are four risk levels, ranging from high+ to low.[162] Each squadron type is evaluated for a risk level and assigned a personnel package based on the identified risk level. As shown in the second column, personnel are embedded either at the

---

[162] High+ squadrons are those squadrons that the Air Force has prioritized for TFTN resources.

squadron level or the group level, providing services to multiple squadrons. Generally speaking, the higher risk the squadron type, the more resources embedded at the squadron level.

Table 5.1. Air Force Mental Health Personnel Packages, by Risk Level

Mental Health Unit Risk Level	Implementation Level	Job Title
High+	Group	Clinical Psychologist
High+	Group	Mental Health Technician
High+	Squadron	Clinical Psychologist
High	Group	Clinical Psychologist
High	Group	Mental Health Technician
High	Squadron	LCSW[a]
Medium	Group	Mental Health Technician
Medium	Squadron	LCSW[a]
Low	Group	Mental Health Technician
Low	Group	LCSW

[a] For squadrons identified as 24-hour operations, an additional LCSW is included for full coverage. This includes aircraft maintenance, missile maintenance, security forces, missile security, logistics readiness, and intelligence squadrons.

Table 5.2. Air Force Physical Health Personnel Packages, by Risk Level

Physical Health Unit Risk Level	Implementation Level	Job Title
High+	Group	Performance Nutritionist
High+	Squadron	Exercise Physiologist
High+	Squadron	Strength and Conditioning Coach
High+	Squadron	Physical Therapist
High+	Squadron	Nutritional Medicine Technician
High	Group	Performance Nutritionist
High	Squadron	Exercise Physiologist
High	Squadron	Strength and Conditioning Coach
High	Squadron	Physical Therapist
Medium	Group	Physical Therapist

In addition to these mental health and physical health personnel packages, the baseline Air Force TFTN implementation plan assumes that religious personnel will be added consistently and steadily on an annual basis and that each installation will receive two program managers and two clinical oversight positions.

Summary of Alternative Courses of Action for Expanding TFTN

Four alternatives or courses of action (COAs) were developed in collaboration with the Air Force TFTN team:

- Baseline: TFTN POM submission with four-year implementation period
- COA 1: modified POM submission assumptions with five-year implementation period
- COA 2: COA 1 assumptions with ten-year implementation period
- COA 3: five-year implementation with personnel reductions in physical health.

We refer to the first COA simply as the baseline. This alternative was the initial Air Force position and is based on the assumptions included in the Air Force–developed FY 2021 POM submission. The remaining COAs are variations on the baseline, including varying the number of years until full implementation, changing the risk level and thus the personnel packages for various squadrons and squadron types, and pushing the implementation of personnel packages from the squadron level to the group level, thus reducing the personnel count included in the implementation.[163]

The following sections provide more-detailed descriptions of each COA. Additionally, the description of the baseline estimate includes all general assumptions made, which are applicable to all of the estimates.

Baseline: TFTN POM Submission with Four-Year Implementation Period

The baseline alternative reflects RAND's cost estimate based on the Air Force implementation assumptions used in their initial POM estimate. Some key differences between the initial RAND cost estimate based on independent RAND assumptions presented in Chapter 4 and the Air Force POM cost estimate are as follows:

- Personnel packages are included for mental health and physical health risk pillars only; personnel packages for social risk are not included in the baseline estimate.
- Religious personnel (chaplains and religious affairs airmen) are included and implemented at a steady rate annually (i.e., not dependent on squadron risk factors).
- Estimates include 1,870 identified squadrons.[164]

---

[163] The basic unit in the Air Force is the squadron. Three or more squadrons typically form a group.

[164] We were able to obtain data for 1,375 squadrons. The Air Force was able to obtain additional data for 495 squadrons and used our model to establish mental and physical health risk for them, for the total of 1,870 squadrons

- Program managers and clinical oversight managers are included on a per-installation basis.

The following ground rules and assumptions are consistent between the independent RAND estimate and the RAND estimate based on Air Force implementation assumptions:

- Costs include only personnel related costs; there are no facilities, equipment, or other non-labor-related costs included.
- All personnel costs are either uniformed military personnel or government civilians; contractors are not included in the estimate. However, the full cost of military personnel and government civilians falls within a wide range of burdened contractor labor costs. Therefore, the cost estimate would be similar if contractor personnel are utilized.
- The cost estimates do not address the potential inability of the government to meet staffing requirements according to the implementation schedule.
- Base military pay, civilian GS pay, BAH, and BAS are all based on the latest FY 2019 rates.
- All other costs are estimated using the OSD CAPE FCoM model, as was used in the cost estimate based on the RAND implementation assumptions discussed in Chapter 4.
- Inflation is included in the estimate according to the OSD FY 2019 "Green Book."

Personnel Type and Pay Grade Assumptions

In addition to the personnel packages identified in Tables 5.1 and 5.2, Table 5.3 summarizes the various types of personnel included in the COA cost estimates. The table lists the assumptions regarding whether a position is assumed to be filled by military personnel (officer or enlisted) or government civilians. Finally, for costing purposes, the pay grade assumptions are included. All civilian pay grades assume a step 5 for costing purposes, whereas officers and enlisted members assume six years and eight years of service, respectively, for costing purposes.

---

that we included in our cost estimates. At the time this was written, the Air Force was considering implementing the TFTN program across the 1,870 squadrons that we included in our estimate.

Table 5.3. Personnel Type and Pay Grade Assumptions for COA Cost Estimates

Job Title	Personnel Type	Pay Grade
Clinical Psychologist	Civilian	GS-14
Mental Health Technician	Enlisted	E-5
Performance Nutritionist	Civilian	GS-13
Licensed Clinical Social Worker	Civilian	GS-12
Exercise Physiologist	Civilian	GS-9
Strength and Conditioning Coach	Civilian	GS-9
Physical Therapist	Officer	O-3
Nutritional Medicine Technician	Enlisted	E-5
Program Manager	Civilian	GS-13
Clinical Oversight	Civilian	GS-13
Chaplain	Officer	O-3
Religious Affairs Airman	Enlisted	E-5

Other Personnel Included in Estimates

As noted previously, the baseline Air Force TFTN implementation plan assumes that religious personnel will be added consistently and steadily on an annual basis. The assumption is that 30 chaplains and 30 religious affairs airmen (of the types identified in Table 5.3) will be added annually for the foreseeable future. The baseline estimate includes these additions for all four years of implementation. However, for the other COAs with longer implementation periods, these additions are included in every year.

Finally, the Air Force TFTN implementation assumes each installation will receive two program managers and two clinical oversight positions (again, of the types identified in Table 5.3). The cost estimate assumes that each installation will receive these positions the first year they receive mental or physical health personnel.

Baseline Cost Estimate Unit Risk Inputs

Table 5.4 details the risk assignments as determined by the Air Force for each unit type for both mental and physical health. The squadron count by unit type is also provided for additional context. Finally, the implementation year is provided in the last column of the table.

Table 5.4. Baseline Mental Health and Physical Health Unit Risk Summary

Unit Type	Squadron Count	Mental Health Risk	Physical Health Risk	Implementation Year
Air Support Operations	15	High+	High+	Year 1
Security Forces Training	1	Medium	Medium	Year 3
Special Operations Aircraft Maintenance	7	Low	Low	Year 4
Aircraft Maintenance	65	High	High	Year 1
Missile Maintenance	5	High	High	Year 2
Security Forces	81	High	High	Year 1
Special Operations Security Force	2	Low	Low	Year 4
Base Defense	3	High	High	Year 2
Missile Security	9	High	High	Year 2
Logistics Readiness	67	High	High	Year 1
Special Operations Logistics Readiness	2	Low	Low	Year 4
Maintenance	49	High	High	Year 1
Special Operations Maintenance	4	Low	Low	Year 4
Civil Engineer	73	High	Medium	Year 2
Special Operations Civil Engineer	2	Low	Low	Year 4
Operations Support	90	High	High	Year 2
Special Operations Support	5	Low	Low	Year 4
Communications	68	High	Medium	Year 2
Special Operations Communications	2	Low	Low	Year 4
Intelligence	51	High	Medium	Year 2
Special Operations Intelligence	2	Low	Low	Year 4
Force Support	75	High	Medium	Year 2
Special Operations Force Support	2	Low	Low	Year 4
Commodities Maintenance	3	High	High	Year 2
Electronics Maintenance	2	High	High	Year 2
Fighter	58	Low	Low	Year 4
Medical Groups[a]	244	Low	Low	Year 4
Reconnaissance	14	Medium	Medium	Year 3
Airlift	33	Medium	Medium	Year 3
Air Mobility	12	Medium	Medium	Year 3
Combat Communications	4	Medium	Medium	Year 3
Air Communications	9	Medium	Medium	Year 3

Unit Type	Squadron Count	Mental Health Risk	Physical Health Risk	Implementation Year
Air Refueling	27	Medium	Medium	Year 3
Air Support	2	Medium	Medium	Year 3
Combat Training	14	Medium	Medium	Year 3
Munitions	21	Medium	Medium	Year 3
Space Operations	6	Medium	Medium	Year 3
Security Support	5	Medium	Medium	Year 3
Training	55	Medium	Medium	Year 3
Other	681	Low	Low	Year 4

a The Medical Groups count is a squadron count; however, personnel packages for Medical Groups are implemented at the group level (71 groups total).

Baseline Cost Estimate and Personnel Count Summary

Table 5.5 summarizes the baseline cost estimate by fiscal year. Each personnel category is summarized by its total annual cost, which is continually increasing as additional personnel are added each year until a year 4 steady state.

Table 5.5. Baseline Cost Estimate

	Year 1 FY 2021	Year 2 FY 2022	Year 3 FY 2023	Year 4 FY 2024
Mental health personnel	$119	$219	$229	$270
Physical health personnel	$126	$189	$199	$204
Religious personnel	$10	$20	$30	$41
Management/oversight personnel	$48	$54	$58	$75
Total annual cost	**$302**	**$482**	**$517**	**$590**

NOTES: All costs are in millions of TY dollars. Some numbers may not sum correctly because of rounding.

Table 5.6 summarizes the baseline personnel count in the same format as the costs shown in Table 5.5. Each personnel category is summarized by its total annual personnel count, which is continually increasing as additional personnel are added each year until a year 4 steady state.

Table 5.6. Baseline Personnel Count

	Year 1 FY 2021	Year 2 FY 2022	Year 3 FY 2023	Year 4 FY 2024
Mental health personnel	839	1,521	1,557	1,807
Physical health personnel	996	1,451	1,487	1,487
Religious personnel	60	120	180	240
Management/oversight personnel	316	348	364	460
Total annual personnel	**2,211**	**3,440**	**3,588**	**3,994**

COA 1: Modified POM Submission with Five-Year Implementation

COA 1 includes the first set of adjustments the Air Force made to the baseline POM estimate. The three major changes are the addition of one year to the implementation schedule, changes to several unit type risk characterizations for both mental and physical health, and changes in year of implementation for several of the unit types. The latter two changes are evident by comparing the baseline mental health and physical health unit risk summary in Table 5.4 with the COA 1 mental health and physical health unit risk summary in Table 5.7.

COA 1 Cost Estimate Unit Risk Inputs

Table 5.7 details the risk assignments as determined by the Air Force for each unit type for both mental and physical health. The squadron count by unit type is also provided for additional context. Finally, the implementation year is provided in the last column of the table.

Table 5.7. COA 1 Mental Health and Physical Health Unit Risk Summary

Unit Type	Squadron Count	Mental Health Risk	Physical Health Risk	Implementation Year
Air Support Operations	15	High+	High+	Year 1
Security Forces Training	1	High	High	Year 1
Special Operations Aircraft Maintenance	7	High	High	Year 1
Aircraft Maintenance	65	High	High	Year 1
Missile Maintenance	5	High	High	Year 1
Security Forces	81	High	High	Year 1
Special Operations Security Force	2	High	High	Year 1
Base Defense	3	High	High	Year 1
Missile Security	9	High	High	Year 1
Logistics Readiness	67	High	High	Year 2
Special Operations Logistics Readiness	2	High	High	Year 2
Maintenance	49	High	High	Year 2
Special Operations Maintenance	4	High	High	Year 2
Civil Engineer	73	High	Medium	Year 3
Special Operations Civil Engineer	2	High	Medium	Year 3
Operations Support	90	High	Low	Year 3
Special Operations Support	5	High	Low	Year 3
Communications	68	High	Medium	Year 3
Special Operations Communications	2	High	Medium	Year 3

Unit Type	Squadron Count	Mental Health Risk	Physical Health Risk	Implementation Year
Intelligence	51	High	Low	Year 3
Special Operations Intelligence	2	High	Low	Year 3
Force Support	75	High	Medium	Year 3
Special Operations Force Support	2	High	Medium	Year 3
Commodities Maintenance	3	High	High	Year 3
Electronics Maintenance	2	High	High	Year 3
Fighter	58	Medium	High	Year 3
Medical Groups[a]	244	High	High	Year 3
Reconnaissance	14	Medium	Medium	Year 4
Airlift	33	Medium	Medium	Year 4
Air Mobility	12	Medium	Medium	Year 4
Combat Communications	4	Medium	Medium	Year 4
Air Communications	9	Medium	Medium	Year 4
Air Refueling	27	Medium	Medium	Year 4
Air Support	2	Medium	Medium	Year 4
Combat Training	14	Medium	Medium	Year 4
Munitions	21	Medium	Medium	Year 4
Space Operations	6	Medium	Low	Year 4
Security Support	5	Medium	Medium	Year 4
Training	55	Medium	Medium	Year 4
Other	681	Low	Low	Year 5

[a] The Medical Groups count is a squadron count; however, personnel packages for Medical Groups are implemented at the group level (71 groups total).

COA 1 Cost Estimate and Personnel Count Summary

Table 5.8 summarizes the COA 1 cost estimate by fiscal year. Each personnel category is summarized by its total annual cost, which is continually increasing as additional personnel are added each year until a year 5 steady state.

Table 5.8. COA 1 Cost Estimate

	Year 1 FY 2021	Year 2 FY 2022	Year 3 FY 2023	Year 4 FY 2024	Year 5 FY 2025
Mental health personnel	$92	$131	$240	$251	$290
Physical health personnel	$93	$142	$214	$226	$230
Religious personnel	$10	$20	$30	$41	$53
Management/oversight personnel	$50	$51	$57	$60	$76
Total annual cost	**$244**	**$344**	**$542**	**$578**	**$649**

NOTES: All costs are in millions of TY dollars. Some numbers may not sum correctly because of rounding.

Table 5.9 summarizes the COA 1 personnel count in the same format as the costs shown in Table 5.8. Each personnel category is summarized by its total annual personnel count, which is continually increasing as additional personnel are added each year until a year 5 steady state.

Table 5.9. COA 1 Personnel Count

	Year 1 FY 2021	Year 2 FY 2022	Year 3 FY 2023	Year 4 FY 2024	Year 5 FY 2025
Mental health personnel	636	908	1,641	1,676	1,904
Physical health personnel	723	1,106	1,619	1,654	1,654
Religious personnel	60	120	180	240	300
Management/oversight personnel	328	328	356	372	460
Total annual personnel	**1,747**	**2,462**	**3,796**	**3,942**	**4,318**

COA 2: Ten-Year Implementation

COA 2 includes almost all of the same assumptions from COA 1 but extends the implementation to ten years in an attempt to reduce the five-year Future Years Defense Program (FYDP) cost by slowing the ramp-up. As shown in the unit risk inputs in Table 5.10, the risk characterizations for each unit type are exactly the same as COA 1, except that the implementation years change to reflect the ten-year implementation.

COA 2 Cost Estimate Unit Risk Inputs

Table 5.10 details the risk assignments as determined by the Air Force for each unit type for both mental and physical health. The squadron count by unit type is also provided for additional context. Finally, the implementation year is provided in the last column of the table.

Table 5.10. COA 2 Mental Health and Physical Health Unit Risk Summary

Unit Type	Squadron Count	Mental Health Risk	Physical Health Risk	Implementation Year
Air Support Operations	15	High+	High+	Year 1
Security Forces Training	1	High	High	Year 1
Special Operations Aircraft Maintenance	7	High	High	Year 2
Aircraft Maintenance	65	High	High	Year 2
Missile Maintenance	5	High	High	Year 2
Security Forces	81	High	High	Year 1
Special Operations Security Force	2	High	High	Year 1
Base Defense	3	High	High	Year 1
Missile Security	9	High	High	Year 1

Unit Type	Squadron Count	Mental Health Risk	Physical Health Risk	Implementation Year
Logistics Readiness	67	High	High	Year 3
Special Operations Logistics Readiness	2	High	High	Year 3
Maintenance	49	High	High	Year 3
Special Operations Maintenance	4	High	High	Year 3
Civil Engineer	73	High	Medium	Year 4
Special Operations Civil Engineer	2	High	Medium	Year 4
Operations Support	90	High	Low	Year 4
Special Operations Support	5	High	Low	Year 5
Communications	68	High	Medium	Year 5
Special Operations Communications	2	High	Medium	Year 5
Intelligence	51	High	Low	Year 5
Special Operations Intelligence	2	High	Low	Year 5
Force Support	75	High	Medium	Year 6
Special Operations Force Support	2	High	Medium	Year 6
Commodities Maintenance	3	High	High	Year 6
Electronics Maintenance	2	High	High	Year 6
Fighter	58	Medium	High	Year 6
Medical Groups[a]	244	High	High	Year 6
Reconnaissance	14	Medium	Medium	Year 7
Airlift	33	Medium	Medium	Year 7
Air Mobility	12	Medium	Medium	Year 7
Combat Communications	4	Medium	Medium	Year 7
Air Communications	9	Medium	Medium	Year 7
Air Refueling	27	Medium	Medium	Year 7
Air Support	2	Medium	Medium	Year 7
Combat Training	14	Medium	Medium	Year 8
Munitions	21	Medium	Medium	Year 8
Space Operations	6	Medium	Low	Year 8
Security Support	5	Medium	Medium	Year 8
Training	55	Medium	Medium	Year 8
Other	681	Low	Low	Years 9 and 10

[a] The Medical Groups count is a squadron count; however, personnel packages for Medical Groups are implemented at the group level (71 groups total).

COA 2 Cost Estimate and Personnel Count Summary

Table 5.11 summarizes the COA 2 cost estimate by fiscal year. Each personnel category is summarized by its total annual cost, which is continually increasing as additional personnel are added each year until a year 10 steady state.

Table 5.11. COA 2 Cost Estimate

	Year 1 FY 2021	Year 2 FY 2022	Year 3 FY 2023	Year 4 FY 2024	Year 5 FY 2025	Year 6 FY 2026	Year 7 FY 2027	Year 8 FY 2028	Year 9 FY 2029	Year 10 FY 2030
Mental health personnel	$54	$94	$134	$190	$228	$256	$265	$273	$303	$322
Physical health personnel	$56	$94	$145	$163	$171	$228	$237	$245	$250	$255
Religious personnel	$10	$20	$30	$41	$53	$65	$77	$90	$103	$117
Management/oversight personnel	$50	$51	$52	$55	$58	$60	$64	$66	$68	$84
Total annual cost	**$170**	**$259**	**$362**	**$450**	**$509**	**$609**	**$643**	**$673**	**$725**	**$779**

NOTES: All costs are in millions of TY dollars. Some numbers may not sum correctly because of rounding.

Table 5.12 summarizes the COA 2 personnel count in the same format as the costs shown in Table 5.11. Each personnel category is summarized by its total annual personnel count, which is continually increasing as additional personnel are added each year until a year 10 steady state.

Table 5.12. COA 2 Personnel Count

	Year 1 FY 2021	Year 2 FY 2022	Year 3 FY 2023	Year 4 FY 2024	Year 5 FY 2025	Year 6 FY 2026	Year 7 FY 2027	Year 8 FY 2028	Year 9 FY 2029	Year 10 FY 2030
Mental health personnel	373	636	908	1,255	1,480	1,641	1,662	1,676	1,830	1,904
Physical health personnel	434	723	1,106	1,197	1,220	1,619	1,640	1,654	1,654	1,654
Religious personnel	60	120	180	240	300	360	420	480	540	600
Management/oversight personnel	328	328	328	340	352	356	372	372	380	460
Total annual personnel	**1,195**	**1,807**	**2,522**	**3,032**	**3,352**	**3,976**	**4,094**	**4,182**	**4,404**	**4,618**

COA 3: Five-Year Implementation with Reductions in Physical Health Personnel

COA 3 returns to the COA 1 implementation schedule of five years, but the major change in this COA is the reduction in physical health personnel. All maintenance and logistics readiness–related squadrons are assumed to receive their respective squadron level personnel packages at the group level rather than embedded at each individual squadron. The impacts of this are evident in the physical health personnel counts in Table 5.13, which are significantly lower than the COA 1 physical health personnel counts in Table 5.7.

COA 3 Cost Estimate Unit Risk Inputs

Table 5.13 details the risk assignments as determined by the Air Force for each unit type for both mental and physical health. The squadron count by unit type is also provided for additional context. Finally, the implementation year is provided in the last column of the table.

Table 5.13. COA 3 Mental Health and Physical Health Unit Risk Summary

Unit Type	Squadron Count	Mental Health Risk	Physical Health Risk	Implementation Year
Air Support Operations	15	High+	High+	Year 1
Security Forces Training	1	High	High	Year 1
Special Operations Aircraft Maintenance	7	High	High	Year 1
Aircraft Maintenance	65	High	High	Year 1
Missile Maintenance	5	High	High	Year 1
Security Forces	81	High	High	Year 1
Special Operations Security Forces	2	High	High	Year 1
Base Defense	3	High	High	Year 1
Missile Security	9	High	High	Year 1
Logistics Readiness	67	High	High	Year 2
Special Operations Logistics Readiness	2	High	High	Year 2
Maintenance	49	High	High	Year 2
Special Operations Maintenance	4	High	High	Year 2
Civil Engineer	73	High	Medium	Year 3
Special Operations Civil Engineer	2	High	Medium	Year 3
Operations Support	90	High	Low	Year 3
Special Operations Support	5	High	Low	Year 3
Communications	68	High	Medium	Year 3
Special Operations Communications	2	High	Medium	Year 3
Intelligence	51	High	Low	Year 3
Special Operations Intelligence	2	High	Low	Year 3
Force Support	75	High	Medium	Year 3
Special Operations Force Support	2	High	Medium	Year 3

Unit Type	Squadron Count	Mental Health Risk	Physical Health Risk	Implementation Year
Commodities Maintenance	3	High	High	Year 3
Electronics Maintenance	2	High	High	Year 3
Fighter	58	Medium	High	Year 3
Medical Groups[a]	244	High	High	Year 3
Reconnaissance	14	Medium	Medium	Year 4
Airlift	33	Medium	Medium	Year 4
Air Mobility	12	Medium	Medium	Year 4
Combat Communications	4	Medium	Medium	Year 4
Air Communications	9	Medium	Medium	Year 4
Air Refueling	27	Medium	Medium	Year 4
Air Support	2	Medium	Medium	Year 4
Combat Training	14	Medium	Medium	Year 4
Munitions	21	Medium	Medium	Year 4
Space Operations	6	Medium	Low	Year 4
Security Support	5	Medium	Medium	Year 4
Training	55	Medium	Medium	Year 4
Other	681	Low	Low	Year 5

[a] The Medical Groups count is a squadron count; however, personnel packages for Medical Groups are implemented at the group level (71 groups total).

COA 3 Cost Estimate and Personnel Count Summary

Table 5.14 summarizes the COA 3 cost estimate by fiscal year. Each personnel category is summarized by its total annual cost, which is continually increasing as additional personnel are added each year until a year 5 steady state.

Table 5.14. COA 3 Cost Estimate

	Year 1	Year 2	Year 3	Year 4	Year 5
	FY 2021	FY 2022	FY 2023	FY 2024	FY 2025
Mental health personnel	$92	$131	$240	$251	$290
Physical health personnel	$74	$80	$149	$159	$162
Religious personnel	$10	$20	$30	$41	$53
Management/oversight personnel	$50	$51	$57	$60	$76
Total annual cost	**$225**	**$281**	**$476**	**$511**	**$581**

NOTES: All costs are in millions of TY dollars. Some numbers may not sum correctly because of rounding.

Table 5.15 summarizes the COA 3 personnel count in the same format as the costs shown in Table 5.14. Each personnel category is summarized by its total annual personnel count, which is continually increasing as additional personnel are added each year until a year 5 steady state.

Table 5.15. COA 3 Personnel Count

	Year 1 FY 2021	Year 2 FY 2022	Year 3 FY 2023	Year 4 FY 2024	Year 5 FY 2025
Mental health personnel	636	908	1,641	1,676	1,904
Physical health personnel	578	611	1,117	1,152	1,152
Religious personnel	60	120	180	240	300
Management/oversight personnel	328	328	356	372	460
Total annual personnel	**1,602**	**1,967**	**3,294**	**3,440**	**3,816**

Comparison of COAs

Cost

Table 5.16 compares the total annual cost based on the cumulative addition of personnel for each of the four alternatives described above. Unsurprisingly, the least expensive option at year 10 is COA 3, because it is the only COA under which personnel are actually reduced. The other three alternatives are more costly at year 10. At year 5, which would encompass the initial FYDP or budgetary period, the least expensive option is COA 2. This is because the implementation is much slower over a ten-year period.

Table 5.16. Comparison of COA Cost Estimates

	Year 1 FY 2021	Year 2 FY 2022	Year 3 FY 2023	Year 4 FY 2024	Year 5 FY 2025	Year 6 FY 2026	Year 7 FY 2027	Year 8 FY 2028	Year 9 FY 2029	Year 10 FY 2030
Baseline	$302	$482	$517	$590	$612	$636	$661	$686	$712	$738
COA 1	$244	$344	$542	$578	$649	$673	$699	$725	$751	$779
COA 2	$170	$259	$362	$450	$509	$609	$643	$673	$725	$779
COA 3	$225	$281	$476	$511	$581	$604	$628	$652	$677	$703

NOTES: All costs are in millions of TY dollars. Some numbers may not sum correctly because of rounding. All cost estimates include 60 religious personnel added annually through year 10.

Timeline

If the Air Force wants to expand quickly, clearly the COAs with the four- or five-year implementation timeline will be preferred. However, such a quick expansion comes at a cost, and with risks, including the risk of not being able to quickly find and hire the number of providers needed to expand the program so quickly. COA 2, with a ten-year implementation timeline, could save costs and allow time to find and hire the number of providers that are needed. However, such a long implementation delays getting embedded resources to units.

Risks

There are risks associated with each of the COAs. As mentioned previously, the COAs with the shorter timelines risk not being able to meet those aggressive timelines for various reasons (including costs and rapid hiring requirements). While the ten-year timeline may seem less risky, such a long timeline could also prevent the expansion from being fully implemented because of changing priorities, budget challenges, etc. Ultimately, the optimal option for expanding TFTN will depend on the Air Force's priorities and goals for TFTN.

Chapter 6. Monitoring the Expansion of Task Force True North

In this chapter, we outline our approach to a framework to monitor the expansion of the TFTN program. We identify issues, metrics, and data collection methods that the monitoring framework should track. Successful implementation of the expansion of TFTN requires that the Air Force develop and continuously maintain a robust monitoring framework and periodically evaluate the impact of policy changes on the strategic goals of TFTN. It is important to note that data collection efforts and implementation monitoring efforts are essentially linked. Data collected for the monitoring framework provide the necessary foundation for the required evaluations. At the same time, the findings from the evaluation studies will inevitably suggest new data elements for the monitoring framework. To assist the Air Force with these essential efforts, in this chapter, we outline elements of a data collection and monitoring framework and describe key characteristics of rigorous evaluation. We also present our sample monitoring framework.

Our Approach to a Monitoring Framework

We organize the issues and measures for our monitoring framework using categories from the Air Force CAF, which are mental, physical, social, and spiritual fitness. We also include types of issues ("What are you measuring?"), measures ("How are you measuring progress, and what information do you need?"), and methods ("How are you collecting the information that you need to measure progress?"). In general, the measures are designed to offer suggestions for ways to track and evaluate those issues that will be monitored; however, there are several ways to measure progress on the expansion of TFTN. We also present several methods for collecting data and discuss the value of considering a variety of methods to measure the different facets of TFTN.

We recommend routine monitoring of the implementation process. However, we recommend that the Air Force also periodically conduct a comprehensive evaluation of the TFTN expansion to reevaluate monitoring priorities. We recommend that an initial evaluation be conducted about three years after implementation and then every five years. Regardless of the outcome of these evaluations, we also emphasize the need for long-term, sustained routine monitoring to identify potential problems quickly as they evolve over time.

Table 6.1 shows the suggested issues, measures, and methods to be monitored during the expansion of TFTN. The Air Force should not consider this list of issues as complete. Instead, the Air Force should consider the list as an initial list. As we stated previously, the evaluation of the expansion of TFTN will present additional issues that the Air Force should monitor and additional data that should be collected.

Potential Data Sources for the Monitoring Framework

The Air Force will need to assess whether it is already collecting the necessary data to monitor the expansion of TFTN, or whether it will need to initiate new data collection efforts. The Air Force can use multiple data sources to develop measures for the issues in our monitoring plan. These data sources include administrative data sources and existing surveys, focus groups, and interviews with stakeholders, including service members, providers, and squadron commanders. Some of the measures are quantitative (including various counts of different incidents and rates), and some of the measures are qualitative in nature. Our monitoring framework is shown in Table 6.1.

Table 6.1. Sample Framework for Monitoring the Expansion of TFTN

	Risks	Measures	Methods
Fitness category: mental	Which AFSCs are most at-risk for suicides?	AFSC suicide rates	Administrative data
	Which squadrons are most at-risk for suicides?	Squadron suicide rates	Administrative data
	What percentage of a squadron has been exposed to combat?	Percentage of a squadron exposed to combat	Administrative data; survey data
	What percentage of a squadron is E1-E4?	Percentage of a squadron that is E1-E4	Administrative data
	What percentage of a squadron has been diagnosed with PTSD?	Percentage of a squadron that has been diagnosed with PTSD	Administrative data
	What percentage of a squadron has been diagnosed with depression?	Percentage of a squadron that has been diagnosed with depression	Administrative data
	What is the command climate like in the squadron?	Assessment of the command climate	Survey, focus group, and interview data; administrative data
	Are airmen utilizing TFTN mental health providers?	Rate of utilization of TFTN mental health providers	Survey, focus group, and interview data
	Has the number of mental health issues decreased in the squadron? Why?	Assessment of the number and cause of mental health issues in the squadron	Administrative data; survey, focus group, and interview data
Fitness category: physical	Which squadrons/AFSCs are most at-risk for physical injuries?	Injury rates	Administrative data
	What percentage of a squadron is nondeployable for physical reasons?	Percentage of a squadron that is non-deployable for physical reasons	Administrative data
	Are airmen utilizing TFTN physical fitness providers?	Rate of utilization of TFTN physical fitness providers	Survey, focus group, and interview data
	Has the number of physical fitness injuries decreased in the squadron? Why?	Assessment of the number and cause of physical fitness injuries in the squadron	Administrative data; survey, focus group, and interview data
Fitness category: social	What is morale like in the squadron?	Assessment of squadron morale	Survey, focus group, and interview data
	What is unit cohesion like in the squadron?	Assessment of squadron unit cohesion	Survey, focus group, and interview data

	Risks	Measures	Methods
	What is the rate of sexual assault in the AFSC?	Sexual assault rate in the AFSC	Administrative data
	What is the rate of sexual assault in the squadron?	Sexual assault rate in the squadron	Administrative data
	What is the rate of misconduct in the squadron?	Rate of misconduct in the squadron	Administrative data
	Are airmen utilizing TFTN social providers?	Rate of utilization of TFTN social providers	Survey, focus group, and interview data
	Has the number of social problems decreased in the squadron? Why?	Assessment of the number and cause of social problems in the squadron	Administrative data; survey, focus group, and interview data
Fitness category: spiritual	Do airmen have adequate access to spiritual advisors?	The Air Force has identified the extent to which Airmen have access to spiritual advisors	Survey, focus group, and interview data
	Do airmen have unmet spiritual needs?	The Air Force has identified any unmet spiritual needs	Survey, focus group, and interview data
	Are airmen utilizing TFTN spiritual providers?	Rate of utilization of TFTN spiritual providers	Survey, focus group, and interview data
Policy issues	Has the Air Force developed a plan for implementing and evaluating TFTN?	The Air Force has developed a plan for implementing and evaluating TFTN	Qualitative review of policy and practices
	Has the Air Force developed a plan for mitigating risks associated with the implementation and evaluations of TFTN?	The Air Force has developed a plan for mitigating risks associated with the implementation and evaluations of TFTN	Qualitative review of policy and practices
	Has the Air Force developed plans for internal and external communications about expanding TFTN?	The Air Force has developed plans for internal and external communications about expanding TFTN	Qualitative review of policy and practices
	Has the Air Force developed a plan for oversight of TFTN and assigned responsibility for oversight?	The Air Force has developed a plan for oversight of TFTN and assigned responsibility for oversight	Qualitative review of policy and practices
	Do all necessary data systems exist to collect data relevant to monitoring implementation of expansion of TFTN?	All necessary data systems exist to collect data relevant to monitoring implementation of expansion of TFTN	Qualitative review of policy and practices
	Do initial budget and resource allocations exist for implementing expansion of TFTN?	Initial budget and resource allocations exist for implementing expansion of TFTN	Qualitative review of policy and practices
Cost and schedule issues	Are actual expenditures consistent with initial budget estimates for the expansion of TFTN?	The Air Force is gathering actual expenditures (labor and non-labor) for implementation of TFTN to update and better inform future cost estimates	Administrative data

Risks	Measures	Methods
Are cost estimate ground rules and assumptions used in budget estimate still consistent with current TFTN implementation plan?	The Air Force updates ground rules and assumptions based on any changes related to TFTN implementation plan	Qualitative review of policy and practices
Are TFTN positions being filled in a timely manner according to implementation schedule?	The Air Force is tracking its ability to fill personnel positions according to the planned implementation schedule	Administrative data

The Need for Evaluation

Establishing and maintaining a monitoring framework is a necessary condition to secure the success of TFTN. But the monitoring framework alone is not sufficient for sustained success of TFTN. For sustained success, we recommend that the Air Force periodically conduct a formal evaluation of TFTN and its impacts on service member fitness and readiness. We recommend that an initial evaluation be conducted about three years after implementation and then every five years. A rigorous evaluation that uses valid and reliable research methods can give the Air Force a formal assessment of the process and outcomes of TFTN.

Conclusion

Monitoring something as sensitive and significant as service member fitness and readiness requires constant vigilance from Air Force leadership and the institution itself. It is not enough to conduct yearly reviews on personnel policies or collect data or statistics. A monitoring plan must consist of long-term and deliberate methods of measuring progress and must include strategies to measure institutional and cultural change over time. This chapter was intended to present and discuss ideas and suggestions for what might be included in such a monitoring framework.

Chapter 7. Recommendations

The planning phase presents the Air Force with a critical window of opportunity to develop strategies, plans, and policies, as well as to put the necessary data systems in place to monitor the expansion of TFTN over time. Insights from other services' experiences with embedded provider programs and the research literature on organizational change inform the following recommendations:[165]

- Ensure top leadership support and commitment.
- Clarify program goals to enable success.
- Plan up front to facilitate data collection and evaluation.
- Consider issues of chain of command and organizational structure.
- Be prepared to respond to changing needs.
- Monitor progress of implementation over time.

Each of these recommendations is discussed in detail below.

Ensure Top Leadership Support and Commitment

Lessons from the other services and the organizational change literature indicate that major organizational change can rarely succeed without leadership support and commitment. The service must ensure that commanders and other unit leaders understand the utility of the TFTN program and that providers are equipped to continually reinforce that message. If top leadership does not reinforce a decision with their continued support and commitment to the expansion of TFTN, expansion may flounder. Senior leaders will also play a critical role in disseminating a consistent message about the expansion of TFTN to both internal and external audiences.

Clarify Program Goals to Enable Success

If a program's purpose and goals are not well articulated, outcomes are impossible to measure. Success of a program is predicated on the foundation that the service must know the program goals and exactly what it wants out of the embedded interactions. Program goals should directly drive how the program should be set up and the principles that govern it. Implementing an embedded health program without a full plan and articulated goals can create problems later. For instance, USSOCOM's original data collection methods were not centralized, which has been challenging both internally and in justifying the program externally.

---

[165] See Kotter (1990), Moran and Brightman (2000), Beckhard and Harris (1987), Van De Ven and Poole (1995), and Cummings and Worley (1993).

Program design, implementation, and evaluation are necessary steps to documenting program effectiveness. It is important to identify metrics that (1) align with program goals, (2) are measurable and reliable, (3) assess implementation progress, and (4) assess program outcomes. A clear evaluation plan will enable program managers to understand and report on program success and monitor the need for programmatic changes.

Plan Up Front to Facilitate Data Collection and Evaluation

Design and implement a standardized data collection process up front so that analysis of program effectiveness and needed changes can be facilitated. Program effectiveness should be tracked over time. The data should also include measures by which effectiveness is assessed. The Navy EMH program has a lack of centralized data and is currently attempting to routinize and centralize some data collection to augment program effectiveness. The Navy is working with different communities within the Navy to identify and record different programs' operations to institutionalize, though not standardize, efforts and lessons learned.

Consider Issues of Chain of Command and Organizational Structure

Chain of command and organizational structure matter, and should be specifically in line with program goals. The Army's EBH team feels that the structure it uses, in which the providers are in the chain of command of the MTF but have a habitual relationship with the unit, is most effective because the provider can provide objective feedback without fear of retribution. In the Navy, line commanders, rather than the MTFs, own the embedded provider billets. Organizational design can affect the degree to which service members are willing to be open with providers (for example, if a provider is in the chain of command, they might be compelled to share sensitive information with the commander, whereas a provider outside the chain of command would not have to).

In addition, centralized program management is needed to create accountability and consistency across the program. Centralized program management of some kind is needed to create responsibility, ensure that the overall mission is matched with the organization that provides the manpower, and create communication and continuity between programs. It is important to note, however, that programs can effectively have both centralized management and tailorable, decentralized implementation. Programs can be tailored to an individual unit's needs so long as there is an overarching goal and program management that ties the programs together. Consider whether centralized management of all programs and increased standardization should be prioritized or whether a more flexible, decentralized model is better given program goals.

Be Prepared to Respond to Changing Needs

Be prepared to iterate and tailor programs to service member needs. The Navy's EMH efforts are not just one program, but rather a collection of programs that have been created based on demand, changing conditions, and lessons learned. OSCAR was originally designed to focus on ground combat units, but over time the Marine Corps noted high demand for embedded care in logistics and aviation career fields and expanded the access accordingly to those communities. Be prepared to tailor the program and iterate as needed, whether by opening the program to different types of units, including additional or different providers, or increasing or decreasing standardization. Supporting the perceived high-risk unit might not be enough, and program managers should be open to expanding embedded care access to other populations and making other program changes based on lessons learned during implementation.

Monitor Progress of Implementation over Time

A strong monitoring plan relies on robust data systems that facilitate the necessary data collection to measure the effectiveness of TFTN. As the Air Force plans for expansion of the TFTN program, it should consider which data systems are already in place to collect the appropriate data to monitor implementation progress over time, and whether any new data systems are necessary.

The monitoring framework presented in Chapter 6 offers the Air Force suggestions on which issues might be included in a monitoring plan, as well as how to measure progress on those issues and what type of data collection methods could be employed. However, for a monitoring plan to be effective, it cannot be static. As data are collected and analyzed, new issues and measures may need to be added to or removed from the monitoring plan. It will also be helpful to identify key measures that leaders should track over time.

Closing Thoughts

As the Air Force begins to think about implementation planning, a critical window of opportunity exists to set in place the strategies, plans, and policies that will guide the implementation process. The Air Force should take full advantage of this opportunity. During this planning process, both near-term and long-term issues should be considered, and the mechanisms put into place during the planning process should be flexible enough to accommodate learning and adjustments. Program implementation will likely be a process of continual, iterative improvements. Putting the systems in place to collect the appropriate data throughout the implementation process will help to build the evidence base for those improvements along the way and will facilitate program success.

Appendix A. Air Force Research Laboratory Profile Risk Score Methodology

According to the 711th HPW, one of the most important factors influencing airmen availability is the number of personnel on profile in a particular unit. "These profiles affect a unit's ability to adequately perform their peacetime or wartime mission. From 1 Jan 2015 through 30 Sep 2018, there were 465,211 distinct mobility or duty restricted profiles for Active Duty Airmen (matched with Air Force Personnel Command data)."[166] The 711th used profile data to determine risk scores for Air Force squadrons in the following way:[167]

Weekly unit profile percentages calculated as

$$P_{Unit} = \frac{Number\ of\ Airmen\ on\ Profile\ During\ Week}{Number\ of\ Airmen\ Assigned\ During\ Week}$$

Weekly Air Force profile percentages are calculated by averaging the weekly unit profile percentages across all ADAF units.

Unit profile (mental health or musculoskeletal injury) risk score is determined by measuring how far it is above or below the Air Force average while accounting for unit size.

This is accomplished by calculating a weekly Z-score:

$$Z_{Unit} = \frac{P_{Unit} - P_{AF}}{\sqrt{P_{AF}(1 - P_{AF})/N_{Unit}}}$$

Over the past 12 months, weighted weekly Z-scores are averaged for each unit (largest weight applied to most recent week). The higher the average, the more time the unit was above the Air Force average across the 12 months.

All units are ordered from positive to negative. Risk group is determined by dividing the units into 20th percentiles. RG1 (highest risk) is the top 20 percent of all the units, RG2 is the second 20th percentile, and so on to RG5.

---

[166] See Erich and Pathak, undated.

[167] See Erich and Pathak, undated.

Appendix B. Semistructured Interview Protocol

1. Could you please describe the EBH model and how it works?
   a. What is the specific purpose of EBH program? E.g., what problems or behaviors does it aim to address?
   b. What is the theory of change?
   c. How long has it been in operation?
2. What type and how many of each provider are part of the embedded team?
3. At what level are the providers embedded (e.g., battalion, company, etc.)?
4. What is the chain of command (direct report to unit commander, belong to the military treatment facility, etc.)?
5. Do providers deploy with teams?
6. Which types, sizes, and echelon of units receive embedded providers?
   a. Are all embedded provider packages the same in terms of number and type of provider?
      i. If not, what different packages exist?
   b. How does the Army determine which units receive the embedded providers?
7. Have you conducted any assessments on the EBH program?
   a. If so, what type, and what were the results?
8. What changes have been made over time to the program as a result of feedback, experience, etc.?
9. What changes do you think need to be made to the program to make it more effective?
10. What advice would you offer to the Air Force as they invest into embedded provider programs?

Abbreviations

AFI	Air Force Instruction
AFRL	Air Force Research Laboratory
AFSC	Air Force Specialty Code
ASIMS	Aeromedical Services Information Management System
BAH	Basic Allowance for Housing
BAS	Basic Allowance for Subsistence
BCT	brigade combat team
BH	behavioral health
BHT	behavioral health technician
CAF	Comprehensive Airman Fitness
CAPE	Cost Assessment and Program Evaluation
COA	course of action
COSC	Combat Operational Stress Control
DoD	U.S. Department of Defense
DOTMLPF-P	doctrine, organization, training, materiel, leadership and education, personnel, facilities, and policy
EBH	Embedded Behavioral Health
EBHT	embedded behavioral health team
EFMP	Exceptional Family Member Program
EMH	Embedded Mental Health
eMHP	embedded Mental Health Program (Navy)
FCoM	Full Cost of Manpower
FY	fiscal year
FYDP	Future Years Defense Program
GS	General Schedule
HPW	Human Performance Wing
LCSW	licensed clinical social worker
MH	mental health
MilPDS	Military Personnel Data System
MLG	marine logistics group
MTF	military treatment facility
NCO	noncommissioned officer
NECC	Navy Expeditionary Combat Command
OSCAR	Operational Stress Control and Readiness
OSD	Office of the Secretary of Defense

OST	operational support team
PH	physical health
PHCoE	Psychological Health Center of Excellence (Defense Health Agency)
POM	Program Objective Memorandum
POTFF	Preservation of the Force and Family
PTSD	posttraumatic stress disorder
SOF	special operations forces
SPRINT	Special Psychiatric Rapid Intervention Team
TFTN	Task Force True North
TY	then year
USSOCOM	U.S. Special Operations Command

References

Acosta, Joie D., Amariah Becker, Jennifer L. Cerully, Michael P. Fisher, Laurie T. Martin, Raffaele Vardavas, Mary Ellen Slaughter, and Terry L. Schell, *Mental Health Stigma in the Military*, Santa Monica, Calif.: RAND Corporation, RR-426-OSD, 2014. As of October 22, 2020:
https://www.rand.org/pubs/research_reports/RR426.html

AFI—*See* Air Force Instruction.

Agerwala, Suneel M., and Elinore F. McCance-Katz, "Integrating Screening, Brief Intervention, and Referral to Treatment (SBIRT) into Clinical Practice Settings: A Brief Review," *Journal of Psychoactive Drugs*, Vol. 44, No. 4, 2012, pp. 307–317.

Air Force Instruction 10-203, *Duty Limiting Conditions*, Washington, D.C.: Department of the Air Force, November 20, 2014.

Air Force Instruction 36-2110, *Total Force Assignments*, Washington, D.C.: Department of the Air Force, October 5, 2018.

Air Force Instruction 36-2907, *Unfavorable Information File (UIF) Program*, Washington, D.C.: Department of the Air Force, November 26, 2014.

Air Force Instruction 90-506, *Comprehensive Airman Fitness*, Washington, D.C.: Department of the Air Force, April 2, 2014.

Air Force Instruction 90-5001, *Integrated Resilience*, Washington, D.C.: Department of the Air Force, January 25, 2019.

American Psychiatric Association, *Diagnostic and Statistical Manual of Mental Disorders, Fifth Edition*, Arlington, Va., 2013.

Army Field Manual No. 4-02.51(8-51), *Combat and Operational Stress Control*, Washington, D.C.: Department of the Army, July 6, 2006.

Army Public Health Center, "Army Injuries, Causes, Risk Factors, and Prevention Overview," webpage, July 30, 2018. As of October 22, 2020:
https://phc.amedd.army.mil/topics/discond/ptsaip/Pages/Army-Injuries-Causes-Risk-Factors-and-Prevention-Overview.aspx

Army Task Force on Behavioral Health, *Corrective Action Plan*, January 2013.

Associated Press, "Rash of Wife Killings at Ft. Bragg Leaves the Base Wondering Why," *New York Times*, July 27, 2002.

Baiocchi, Dave, *Measuring Army Deployments to Iraq and Afghanistan*, Santa Monica, Calif.: RAND Corporation, RR-145-A, 2013. As of October 22, 2020: https://www.rand.org/pubs/research_reports/RR145.html

Beckhard, Richard, and Reuben T. Harris, *Organizational Transitions: Managing Complex Change*, 2nd ed., Reading, Mass.: Addison-Wesley, 1987.

Carabajal, Shannon, "Army Expanding Successful Embedded Behavioral Health Program," Army.mil, November 17, 2011. As of October 22, 2020: https://www.army.mil/article/69479/army_expanding_successful_embedded_behavioral_heal th_program

Carey, Lindsay B., and Timothy J. Hodgson, "Chaplaincy, Spiritual Care and Moral Injury: Considerations Regarding Screening and Treatment," *Frontiers in Psychiatry*, Vol. 9, December 5, 2018.

Carey, Lindsay B., Timothy J. Hodgson, Lillian Krikheli, Rachel Y. Soh, Annie-Rose Armour, Taranjeet K. Singh, and Cassandra G. Impiombato, "Moral Injury, Spiritual Care and the Role of Chaplains: An Exploratory Scoping Review of Literature and Resources," *Journal of Religion and Health*, Vol. 55, 2016, pp. 1218–1245.

Chairman of the Joint Chiefs of Staff Instruction 3405.01, *Chairman's Total Force Fitness Framework*, September 1, 2011.

Chief of Naval Operations, OPNAV Instruction 6520.1A, *Operational Stress Control Program*, Washington, D.C.: Department of the Navy, June 14, 2016.

Cho-Stutler, Laura, "Staff Voices: Q & A on the Army's Embedded Behavioral Health (EBH) Program," online interview with Kay Beaulieu, a psychologist in the Public Health Service, blog of the Uniformed Services University's Center for Deployment Psychology, October 7, 2013. As of October 22, 2020: https://deploymentpsych.org/blog/staff-voices-q-army%e2%80%99s-embedded-behavioral-health-ebh-program

Commander, Navy Expeditionary Combat Command, and Commander, Navy Expeditionary Combat Command Pacific, COMNECC/COMNECCPAC Instruction 1754.1C, *Family Readiness Program*, Washington, D.C.: Department of the Navy, January 8, 2015.

Connor, Kathryn M., Jonathan R. T. Davidson, and Li-Ching Lee, "Spirituality, Resilience, and Anger in Survivors of Violent Trauma: A Community Survey," *Journal of Traumatic Stress*, Vol. 16, No. 5, October 2003, pp. 487–494.

Crum-Cianflone, Nancy F., and Isabel Jacobson, "Gender Differences of Postdeployment Post-Traumatic Stress Disorder Among Service Members and Veterans of the Iraq and Afghanistan Conflicts," *Epidemiologic Reviews*, Vol. 36, 2014, pp. 5–18.

Cummings, Thomas G., and Christopher G. Worley, *Organization Development and Change*, 5th edition, St. Paul, Minn.: West Publishing Co., 1993.

Damen, Annelieke, Carmen Schuhmann Leget, Carlo Leget, and George Fitchett, "Can Outcome Research Respect the Integrity of Chaplaincy? A Review of Outcome Studies," *Journal of Health Care Chaplaincy*, Vol. 26, No. 4, 2020, pp. 131–158.

Department of Defense Instruction 6025.19, *Individual Medical Readiness*, Washington, D.C.: U.S. Department of Defense, June 9, 2014.

Department of Defense Instruction 6490.12, *Mental Health Assessments for Service Members Deployed in Connection with a Contingency Operation*, Washington, D.C.: U.S. Department of Defense, February 26, 2013.

DiBenigno, Julia, *Command-Provider Relationships in Embedded Behavioral Health*, Cambridge, Mass.: Massachusetts Institute of Technology, 2016. As of November 3, 2020: https://dspace.mit.edu/handle/1721.1/102544

DoD—*See* U.S. Department of Defense.

DODI—*See* Department of Defense Instruction.

DSM-5—*See* American Psychiatric Association, *Diagnostic and Statistical Manual of Mental Disorders, Fifth Edition*, Arlington, Va., 2013.

Elnitsky, Christine A., Michael P. Fisher, and Cara L. Blevins, "Military Service Member and Veteran Reintegration: A Conceptual Analysis, Unified Definition, and Key Domains," *Frontiers in Psychology*, Vol. 8, 2017.

Engel Charles C., Thomas Oxman, Christopher Yamamoto, Darin Gould, Sheila Barry, Patrice Stewart, Kurt Kroenke, John W. Williams Jr., and Allen J. Dietrich, "RESPECT-Mil: Feasibility of a Systems-Level Collaborative Care Approach to Depression and Post-Traumatic Stress Disorder in Military Primary Care," *Military Medicine*, Vol. 173, No. 10, October 2008, pp. 935–940.

Erich, Roger, and Sonal Pathak, "Mental Health and MSKI Risk Score Generation Using ASIMS Profile Data," PowerPoint presentation, undated.

Executive Order 13426, *Establishing a Commission on Care for America's Returning Wounded Warriors and a Task Force on Returning Global War on Terror Heroes*, Washington, D.C.: The White House, March 6, 2007.

Faison, C. Forrest, III, *Statement of Vice Admiral C. Forrest Faison III, MC, USN, Surgeon General of the Navy, Before the Subcommittee on Defense of the Senate Committee on Appropriations, Subject: Defense Health Program*, April 26, 2018.

Foa, Edna B., Diana Hearst-Ikeda, and Kevin J. Perry, "Evaluation of a Brief Cognitive-Behavioral Program for the Prevention of Chronic PTSD in Recent Assault Victims," *Journal of Consulting and Clinical Psychology*, Vol. 63, No. 6, 1995, pp. 948–955.

Frank, Christine, Mark A. Zamorski, Jennifer E. C. Lee, and Ian Colman, "Deployment-Related Trauma and Post-Traumatic Stress Disorder: Does Gender Matter?" *European Journal of Psychotraumatology*, Vol. 9, No. 1, 2018.

Headquarters, U.S. Army, *Executive Order 236-12: Army Implementation of Behavioral Health System of Care (BHSOC) Embedded Behavioral Health*, Washington, D.C., July 2012.

Hoge, Charles W., Jennifer L. Auchterlonie, and Charles S. Milliken, "Mental Health Problems, Use of Mental Health Services, and Attrition from Military Service After Returning from Deployment to Iraq or Afghanistan," *Journal of the American Medical Association*, Vol. 295, No. 9, 2006, pp. 1023–1032.

Hoge, Charles W., Carl A. Castro, Stephen C. Messer, Dennis McGurk, Dave I. Cotting, and Robert L. Koffman, "Combat Duty in Iraq and Afghanistan, Mental Health Problems, and Barriers to Care," *New England Journal of Medicine*, Vol. 351, 2004, pp. 13–22.

Hoge, Charles W., Christopher G. Ivany, Edward A. Brusher, Millard D. Brown III, John C. Shero, Amy B. Adler, Christopher H. Warner, and David T. Orma, "Transformation of Mental Health Care for U.S. Soldiers and Families During the Iraq and Afghanistan Wars: Where Science and Politics Intersect," *American Journal of Psychiatry*, Vol. 173, No. 4, 2015, pp. 334–343.

Hoge, Charles W., Artin Terhakopian, Carl A. Castro, Stephen C. Messer, and Charles C. Engel, "Association of Posttraumatic Stress Disorder with Somatic Symptoms, Health Care Visits, and Absenteeism Among Iraq War Veterans," *American Journal of Psychiatry*, Vol. 164, No. 1, 2007, pp. 150–153.

Holstein, Peter, "Operational Support Teams Work Inside 'Beating Heart' of Air Force," Air Force News, September 12, 2018. As of October 22, 2020:
https://www.af.mil/News/Article-Display/Article/1628702/operational-support-teams-work-inside-beating-heart-of-air-force/

Institute of Medicine, *Preventing Psychological Disorders in Service Members and Their Families: An Assessment of Programs*, Washington, D.C.: The National Academies Press, 2014.

Kade, Harold Dennis, "Navy Expeditionary Combat Command embedded Mental Health Program (eMHP) IdeaFest: Hampton Roads Innovation Case Study," PowerPoint presentation, July 31, 2013.

Koffman, Robert L., Richard D. Bergthold, Justin S. Campbell, Richard J. Westphal, Paul Hammer, Thomas A. Gaskin, John Ralph, Edward Simmer, and William P. Nash, "Expeditionary Operational Stress Control in the US Navy," in Army Medical Department, Borden Institute, *Combat and Operational Behavioral Health*, 2006.

Kotter, John P., *A Force for Change: How Leadership Differs from Management*, New York: Free Press, 1990.

Koufas, Ted, Program Executive Officer for Services, "NDIA Breakfast," PowerPoint presentation, October 11, 2016.

MacGregor, Andrew J., Janet J. Tang, Amber L. Dougherty, and Michael R. Galarneau, "Deployment-Related Injury and Posttraumatic Stress Disorder in U.S. Military Personnel," *Injury*, Vol. 44, No. 11, 2013, pp. 1458–1464.

Marquis, Jefferson P., Coreen Farris, Kimberly Curry Hall, Kristy N. Kamarck, Nelson Lim, Douglas Shontz, Paul S. Steinberg, Robert Stewart, Thomas E. Trail, Jennie W. Wenger, Anny Wong, and Eunice C. Wong, *Improving Oversight and Coordination of Department of Defense Programs That Address Problematic Behaviors Among Military Personnel: Final Report*, Santa Monica, Calif.: RAND Corporation, RR-1352-OSD, 2017. As of October 22, 2020:
https://www.rand.org/pubs/research_reports/RR1352.html

Mayo, Jonathan A., Andrew J. MacGregor, Amber L. Dougherty, and Michael R. Galarneau, "Role of Occupation on New-Onset Post-Traumatic Stress Disorder and Depression Among Deployed Military Personnel," *Military Medicine*, Vol. 178, No. 9, 2013, pp. 945–950.

McRaven, William H., *Posture Statement of Admiral William H. McRaven, USN Commander, United States Special Operations Command Before the 112th Congress Senate Armed Services Committee*, 2012.

Meadows, Sarah O., Charles C. Engel, Rebecca L. Collins, Robin L. Beckman, Matthew Cefalu, Jennifer Hawes-Dawson, Molly Waymouth, Amii M. Kress, Lisa Sontag-Padilla, Rajeev Ramchand, and Kayla M. Williams, *2015 Health Related Behaviors Survey: Health Promotion and Disease Prevention Among U.S. Active-Duty Service Members*, Santa Monica, Calif.: RAND Corporation, RB-9955/2-OSD, 2018a. As of October 22, 2020: https://www.rand.org/pubs/research_briefs/RB9955z2.html

Meadows, Sarah O., Charles C. Engel, Rebecca L. Collins, Robin L. Beckman, Matthew Cefalu, Jennifer Hawes-Dawson, Molly Waymouth, Amii M. Kress, Lisa Sontag-Padilla, Rajeev Ramchand, and Kayla M. Williams, *Are They Living Healthy? How Well Are Airmen Taking Care of Themselves*, Santa Monica, Calif.: RAND Corporation, IG-129/1, 2018b. As of October 22, 2020:
https://www.rand.org/pubs/infographics/IG129z1.html

Meredith, Lisa S., Cathy D. Sherbourne, Sarah J. Gaillot, Lydia Hansell, Hans V. Ritschard, Andrew M. Parker, and Glenda Wrenn, *Promoting Psychological Resilience in the U.S. Military*, Santa Monica, Calif.: RAND Corporation, MG-996-OSD, 2011. As of October 22, 2020:
https://www.rand.org/pubs/monographs/MG996.html

Miletich, Derek, "COMSUBPAC embedded Mental Health Program (eMHP)," Submarine Force Pacific *SUBPAC Spotlight* blog, March 13, 2017. As of November 3, 2020:
https://www.csp.navy.mil/Blog/Blog-Post/Article/1113830/comsubpac-embedded-mental-health-program-emhp/

Moran, John W., and Baird K. Brightman, "Leading Organizational Change," *Journal of Workplace Learning*, Vol. 12, No. 2, 2000, pp. 66–74.

Morral, Andrew R., Kristie L. Gore, and Terry L. Schell, eds., *Sexual Assault and Sexual Harassment in the U.S. Military: Volume 2. Estimates for Department of Defense Service Members from the 2014 RAND Military Workplace Study*, Santa Monica, Calif.: RAND Corporation, RR-870/2-1-OSD, 2015. As of October 22 2020:
https://www.rand.org/pubs/research_reports/RR870z2-1.html

Morral, Andrew R., Kristie L. Gore, and Terry L. Schell, eds., *Sexual Assault and Sexual Harassment in the U.S. Military: Evaluating Estimates from the 2014 RAND Military Workplace Study*, Santa Monica, Calif.: RAND Corporation, RB-9899-OSD, 2016. As of October 26, 2020:
https://www.rand.org/pubs/research_briefs/RB9899.html

Morral, Andrew R., Kristie Gore, Terry L. Schell, Barbara Bicksler, Coreen Farris, Bonnie Ghosh-Dastidar, Lisa H. Jaycox, Dean Kilpatrick, Steve Kistler, Amy Street, et al., *Sexual Assault and Sexual Harassment in the U.S. Military: Highlights from the 2014 RAND Military Workplace Study*, Santa Monica, Calif.: RAND Corporation, RB-9841-OSD, 2015.

Morral, Andrew R., Terry L. Schell, Matthew Cefalu, Jessica Hwang, and Andrew Gelman, *Sexual Assault and Sexual Harassment in the U.S. Military Volume 5. Estimates for Installation- and Command-Level Risk of Sexual Assault and Sexual Harassment from the 2014 RAND Military Workplace Study*, Santa Monica, Calif.: RAND Corporation, RR-870/7-OSD, 2018. As of October 22, 2020:
https://www.rand.org/pubs/research_briefs/RB9841.html

Morral, Andrew R., Terry L. Schell, Matthew Cefalu, Jessica Hwang, and Andrew Gelman, *Sexual Assault and Sexual Harassment in the U.S. Military: Annex to Volume 5. Tabular Results from the 2014 RAND Military Workplace Study for Installation- and Command-Level Risk of Sexual Assault and Sexual Harassment*, Santa Monica, Calif.: RAND Corporation,

RR-870/8-OSD, 2018. As of October 22, 2020:
https://www.rand.org/pubs/research_reports/RR870z8.html

Nash, William P., *US Marine Corps and Navy Combat and Operational Stress Continuum Model: A Tool for Leaders*, in Army Medical Department, Borden Institute, *Combat and Operational Behavioral Health*, 2006.

Naval Center for Combat and Operational Stress Control, "Resilience and Mental Health: U.S. Marine Corps and U.S. Navy Combat & Operational Stress Control," July 2013. As of November 3, 2020:
http://www.workplacementalhealth.org/Case-Studies/Naval-Center-for-Combat-Operational-Stress-Control

Navy Medical Forces Atlantic, "Special Psychiatric Rapid Intervention Team," undated. As of November 3, 2020:
https://www.med.navy.mil/sites/nme/SitePages/sprint.aspx

Negrusa, Sebastian, Brighita Negrusa, and James Hosek, "Gone to War: Have Deployments Increased Divorces?" *Journal of Popular Economics*, Vol. 27, No. 2, 2014, pp. 473–496.

Nindl, Bradley C., Thomas J. Williams, Patricia A. Deuster, Nikki L. Butler, and Bruce H. Jones, "Strategies for Optimizing Military Physical Readiness and Preventing Musculoskeletal Injuries in the 21st Century," *U.S. Army Medical Department Journal*, October–December 2013, pp. 5–23.

Office of the Under Secretary of Defense (Comptroller), *National Defense Budget Estimates for FY 2019*, April 2018.

Office of the Secretary of Defense, Cost Assessment and Program Evaluation, "Full Cost of Manpower (FCoM)," website, 2020, Not available to the general public. As of November 3, 2020:
https://fcom.cape.osd.mil/user/default.aspx

Pierce, Katherine E., David Broderick, Scott Johnston, and Kathryn J. Holloway, "Embedded Mental Health in the United States Marine Corps," *Military Medicine*, Vol. 185, Nos. 9–10, September–October 2020.

Pietrzak, Robert H., Risë B. Goldstein, Steven M. Southwick, and Bridget F. Grant, "Prevalence and Axis I Comorbidity of Full and Partial Posttraumatic Stress Disorder in the United States: Results from Wave 2 of the National Epidemiologic Survey on Alcohol and Related Conditions," *Journal of Anxiety Disorders*, Vol. 25, No. 3, April 2011, pp. 456–465.

President's Commission on Care for America's Returning Wounded Warriors, *Serve, Support, Simplify: Report of the President's Commission on Care for America's Returning Wounded*

Warriors, July 2007. As of October 22, 2020:
http://www.patriotoutreach.org/docs/presidents-commission-report-july-2007.pdf

Psychological Health Center of Excellence, "Posttraumatic Stress Disorder (PTSD)," webpage, undated-a. As of October 22. 2020:
https://www.pdhealth.mil/clinical-guidance/clinical-conditions/posttraumatic-stress-disorder-ptsd

Psychological Health Center of Excellence, "Suicide Risk Resources for Providers," webpage, undated-b. As of October 22. 2020:
https://www.pdhealth.mil/clinical-guidance/clinical-conditions/suicide-risk

Ramchand, Rajeev, Rena Rudavsky, Sean Grant, Terri Tanielian, and Lisa Jaycox, "Prevalence of, Risk Factors for, and Consequences of Posttraumatic Stress Disorder and Other Mental Health Problems in Military Populations Deployed to Iraq and Afghanistan," *Current Psychiatry Reports*, Vol. 17, No. 5, 2015.

Ramchand, Rajeev, Sangeeta C. Ahluwalia, Lea Xenakis, Eric Apaydin, Laura Raaen, and Geoffrey Grimm, "A Systematic Review of Peer-Supported Interventions for Health Promotion and Disease Prevention," *Preventive Medicine*, Vol. 101, August 2017, pp. 156–170.

Robinson, Col, AF/A1/A1Z, *Bullet Background Paper on FY21 True North Expansion Funded Via PEC 88737F*, January 22, 2019a.

Robinson, Col, AF/A1/A1Z, *Talking Paper on FY21 True North Expansion Via PEC 88737F*, January 22, 2019b.

Schnurr, Paula P., Carol A. Lunney, Michelle J. Bovin, and Brian P. Marx, "Posttraumatic Stress Disorder and Quality of Life: Extension of Findings to Veterans of the Wars in Iraq and Afghanistan," *Clinical Psychology Review*, Vol. 29, No. 8, December 2009, pp. 727–735.

Sharma, Vanshdeep, Deborah B. Marin, Harold K. Koenig, Adriana Feder, Brian M. Iacoviello, Steven M. Southwick, and Robert H. Pietrzak, "Religion, Spirituality, and Mental Health of U.S. Military Veterans: Results from the National Health and Resilience in Veterans Study," *Journal of Affective Disorders*, Vol. 217, August 2017, pp. 197–204.

Shenbergerhess, Ashley, "Dolphin Docs: Mental Health Providers Embedded in the Submarine Community," Psychological Health Center of Excellence, *Clinician's Corner Blog*, January 7, 2019.

Smith, Stacy, "Exploring the Interaction of Trauma and Spirituality," *Traumatology*, Vol. 10, No. 4, 2004, pp. 231–243.

Smith, Tyler C., Margaret A. K. Ryan, Deborah L. Wingard, Donald J. Slymen, James F. Sallis, and Donna Kritz-Silverstein, for the Millennium Cohort Study Team, "New Onset and

Persistent Symptoms of Post-Traumatic Stress Disorder Self Reported After Deployment and Combat Exposures: Prospective Population Based U.S. Military Cohort Study," *BMJ*, February 16, 2008.

Srinivasan, Jayakanth, *Lessons Learned from Implementing Embedded Behavioral Health at Four Army Installations*, Cambridge, Mass.: Massachusetts Institute of Technology, 2016a. As of November 3, 2020:
https://dspace.mit.edu/handle/1721.1/102561

Srinivasan, Jayakanth, *Preliminary Evidence on the Effectiveness of Embedded Behavioral Health*, Cambridge, Mass.: Massachusetts Institute of Technology, 2016b. As of November 3, 2020:
https://dspace.mit.edu/handle/1721.1/102562

Srinivasan, Jayakanth, and Julia DiBenigno, *Developing the Embedded Behavioral Health Checklists*, Cambridge, Mass.: Massachusetts Institute of Technology, Sociotechnical Systems Research Center, November 20, 2014. As of November 3, 2020:
http://hdl.handle.net/1721.1/102554

Teyhen, Deydre S., Scott W. Shaffer, Robert J. Butler, Stephen L. Goffar, Kyle B. Kiesel, Daniel I. Rhon, Jared N. Williamson, and Phillip J. Plisky, "What Risk Factors Are Associated with Musculoskeletal Injury in US Army Rangers? A Prospective Prognostic Study," *Clinical Orthopaedics and Related Research*, Vol. 473, No. 9, 2015, pp. 2948–2958.

USAF Services, "Exceptional Family Member Program/Special Needs," undated. As of November 3, 2020:
https://www.usafservices.com/Home/SpouseSupport/SpecialNeeds.aspx

U.S. Air Force, *Task Force-True North Charter*, December 21, 2016.

U.S. Air Force, *Performance Work Statement (PWS), Task Force True North (TFTN), Resiliency and Prevention Support Contract*, posted date October 5, 2017. Accessed from GovTribe website, as of July 25, 2022:
https://govtribe.com/opportunity/federal-contract-opportunity/task-force-true-north-fa701417r1016#

U.S. Army Medical Command, *Operational Order 12-63: Embedded Behavioral Health Team Implementation*, August 17, 2012.

U.S. Army Medical Command, *Embedded Behavioral Health Guide*, MEDCOM Pamphlet No. 40-19, Fort Sam Houston, Tex.: Headquarters, U.S. Army Medical Command, October 10, 2014.

U.S. Army Medical Command, Fragmentary Order 5 to *Operational Order 12-63: Embedded Behavioral Health Team Implementation*, 2015.

U.S. Department of Defense, *Department of Defense Plan to Achieve the Vision of the DoD Task Force on Mental Health: Report to Congress*, Washington, D.C., September 2007.

U.S. Department of Health and Human Services, Office of Disease Prevention and Health Promotion, "Healthy People 2020," website, 2020. As of November 5, 2020: https://www.healthypeople.gov/2020/

U.S. Department of Veterans Affairs and U.S. Department of Defense, *VA/DoD Clinical Practice Guideline for the Management of Posttraumatic Stress Disorder and Acute Stress Disorder*, 2017. As of April 29, 2019: https://www.healthquality.va.gov/guidelines/MH/ptsd/VADoDPTSDCPGFinal012418.pdf

U.S. Department of Veterans Affairs and U.S. Department of Defense, *VA/DoD Clinical Practice Guideline for Assessment and Management of Patients at Risk for Suicide*, June 2013.

U.S. Department of Veterans Affairs and U.S. Department of Defense, *VA/DoD Clinical Practice Guideline for Management of Major Depressive Disorders*, 2016.

U.S. Department of Veterans Affairs and U.S. Department of Defense, *VA/DoD Clinical Practice Guideline for Management of Substance Use Disorder (SUD)*, 2015.

U.S. Marine Corps, *Combat and Operational Stress Control*, Marine Corps Reference Publication (MCRP) 6-11C/Navy Tactics, Techniques, and Procedures (NTTP 1-15M), December 20, 2010.

U.S. Marine Corps, *Operational Stress Control and Readiness Training Guidance*, MARADMINS 597/11, October 7, 2011.

U.S. Marine Corps, *Combat and Operational Stress Control Program*, Marine Corps Order 5351.1, February 22, 2013.

U.S. Navy Chaplain Corps, "Spiritual Fitness Guide," May 2, 2012. As of July 25, 2022: https://www.iimef.marines.mil/Portals/1/documents/PWYE/Toolkit/MAPIT-Modules/Marine-Fitness/SpiritualFitnessGuide.pdf?ver=2018-01-23-133357-223

U.S. Navy, Director, 21st Century Sailor Office (N17), *Command Resilience Team Guide*, Washington, D.C.: Department of the Navy, June 26, 2018.

USSOCOM—*See* U.S. Special Operations Command.

U.S. Special Operations Command, "About POTFF: About USSOCOM Preservation of the Force and Family (POTFF)," webpage, February 13, 2019a. As of November 3, 2020: https://www.socom.mil/POTFF/Pages/About-POTFF.aspx

U.S. Special Operations Command, *Performance Work Statement (PWS), Preservation of the Force and Family (POTFF) Programs Support Contract*, March 12, 2018. Available at

Government Contracts and Bids website, accessed May 6, 2019b: https://www.govcb.com/government-bids/POTFF-NBD00159911946519268.htm

U.S. Special Operations Command, "Preservation of the Force and Family (POTFF) Mission," webpage, undated. Accessed April 8, 2019: https://www.socom.mil/ussocom-enterprise/hq

VA and DoD—*See* U.S. Department of Veterans Affairs and U.S. Department of Defense.

Van De Ven, Andrew H., and Marshall Scott Poole, "Explaining Development and Change in Organizations," *Academy of Management: The Academy of Management Review*, Vol. 20, No. 3, July 1995, pp. 510–540.

Vaughan, Christine Anne, Carrie M. Farmer, Joshua Breslau, and Crystal Burnette, *Evaluation of the Operational Stress Control and Readiness (OSCAR) Program*, Santa Monica, Calif.: RAND Corporation, RR-562-OSD, 2015. As of October 22, 2020: https://www.rand.org/pubs/research_reports/RR562.html

Weinick, Robin M., Ellen Burke Beckjord, Carrie M. Farmer, Laurie T. Martin, Emily M. Gillen, Joie D. Acosta, Michael P. Fisher, Jeffrey Garnett, Gabriella C. Gonzalez, Todd C. Helmus, Lisa H. Jaycox, Kerry Reynolds, Nicholas Salcedo, and Deborah M. Scharf, *Programs Addressing Psychological Health and Traumatic Brain Injury Among U.S. Military Servicemembers and Their Families*, Santa Monica, Calif.: RAND Corporation, TR-950-OSD, 2011. As of October 22, 2020: https://www.rand.org/pubs/technical_reports/TR950.html

Wood, Dennis Patrick, Robert L. Koffman, and Anthony A. Arita, "Psychiatric Medevacs During a 6-Month Aircraft Carrier Battle Group Deployment to the Persian Gulf: A Navy Force Health Protection Preliminary Report," *Military Medicine*, Vol. 168, No. 1, January 2003, pp. 43–47.

Ziemke, Gregg W., Robert L. Koffman, and Dennis Patrick Wood, "'Tip of the Spear' Physical Therapy During a 6-Month Deployment to the Persian Gulf: A Preliminary Report," *Military Medicine*, Vol. 166, No. 6, 2001, pp. 505–509.